DEMYSTIFYING
SCHIZOPHRENIA

for the General Practitioner

Steven J. Siegel, MD, PhD
Associate Professor
Department of Psychiatry
Director
Translational Neuroscience Program
University of Pennsylvania
Philadelphia, PA

LaRiena N. Ralph, BS
Clinical Coordinator
Neuropsychiatric Clinic at Penn Behavioral Health
University of Pennsylvania
Philadelphia, PA

JONES AND BARTLETT PUBLISHERS
Sudbury, Massachusetts
BOSTON   TORONTO   LONDON   SINGAPORE

World Headquarters

Jones and Bartlett Publishers	Jones and Bartlett Publishers	Jones and Bartlett Publishers
40 Tall Pine Drive	Canada	International
Sudbury, MA 01776	6339 Ormindale Way	Barb House, Barb Mews
978-443-5000	Mississauga, Ontario L5V 1J2	London W6 7PA
info@jbpub.com	Canada	United Kingdom
www.jbpub.com		

Jones and Bartlett's books and products are available through most bookstores and online booksellers. To contact Jones and Bartlett Publishers directly, call 800-832-0034, fax 978-443-8000, or visit our website, www.jbpub.com.

Substantial discounts on bulk quantities of Jones and Bartlett's publications are available to corporations, professional associations, and other qualified organizations. For details and specific discount information, contact the special sales department at Jones and Bartlett via the above contact information or send an email to specialsales@jbpub.com.

The authors, editor, and publisher have made every effort to provide accurate information. However, they are not responsible for errors, omissions, or for any outcomes related to the use of the contents of this book and take no responsibility for the use of the products and procedures described. Treatments and side effects described in this book may not be applicable to all people; likewise, some people may require a dose or experience a side effect that is not described herein. Drugs and medical devices are discussed that may have limited availability controlled by the Food and Drug Administration (FDA) for use only in a research study or clinical trial. Research, clinical practice, and government regulations often change the accepted standard in this field. When consideration is being given to use of any drug in the clinical setting, the healthcare provider or reader is responsible for determining FDA status of the drug, reading the package insert, and reviewing prescribing information for the most up-to-date recommendations on dose, precautions, and contraindications, and determining the appropriate usage for the product. This is especially important in the case of drugs that are new or seldom used.

Production Credits
Sr. Acquisitions Editor: Alison Hankey
Sr. Editorial Assistant: Jessica Acox
Production Editor: Daniel Stone
Marketing Manager: Alisha Weisman
V.P., Manufacturing and Inventory Control: Therese Connell
Composition: Auburn Associates, Inc.
Printing and Binding: Malloy, Inc.
Cover Printing: Malloy, Inc.
Cover Design: Kristin Parker
Cover image: © Loongar/Dreamstime.com

Library of Congress Cataloging-in-Publication Data
Siegel, Steven J.
    Demystifying schizophrenia for the general practitioner / Steven J. Siegel, LaRiena Ralph.
        p. ; cm.
    Includes bibliographical references and index.
    ISBN-13: 978-0-7637-5865-3
    ISBN-10: 0-7637-5865-5
    1. Schizophrenia. I. Ralph, LaRiena. II. Title.
    [DNLM: 1. Schizophrenia—diagnosis. 2. Schizophrenia—physiopathology.
3. Schizophrenia—therapy. WM 203 S571d 2010]
    RC514.S5435 2010
    616.89′8—dc22

                                                                                        2009019551

6048

Printed in the United States of America
13 12 11 10 09   10 9 8 7 6 5 4 3 2 1

Table of Contents

Preface

Schizophrenia is among the most devastating of all illnesses, affecting approximately 1–2% of the world's population. The onset for this disorder is generally between 20 and 30 years of age, with a chronic, unremitting disease course for the duration of the patient's life. Schizophrenia is characterized by two main symptom clusters, positive symptoms and negative symptoms, as well as lasting cognitive and functional disabilities.

Positive symptoms include hallucinations, delusions, and disorganized, often bizarre thoughts and behavior. Positive symptoms refer to symptoms that most individuals do not normally experience, whereas **negative symptoms** are considered to be the loss or absence of normal traits or abilities. Negative symptoms include loss of interest and motivation, as well as loss of normal ability to both feel and express emotion. Lasting functional decline is a hallmark of the illness leading to the enormous personal, familial, and societal costs caused by disability and lost productivity.

This book addresses historical and current understanding and approaches to the clinical presentation, pathophysiology, and treatment of schizophrenia. Although schizophrenia remains among the most severe and debilitating illnesses known to medicine, its treatment has remained virtually unchanged for over 50 years due to the lack of significant advances in our understanding of its neurological underpinnings or pharmacological targets.

Various aspects of the presentation, manifestation, and treatment of schizophrenia are discussed using clinical vignettes and case presentations. Differential diagnosis, comorbid conditions, and complications relevant to nonpsychiatry specialties are illustrated. The book discusses several promising areas for future therapeutic advances, including improved drug delivery strategies that have the potential to effect rapid and dramatic improvements in schizophrenia outcomes.

Acknowledgments

Steve Siegel
I would like to thank my family, Ayuko, Sarah, & Jona, for their support and patience throughout the 2 years of nights and weekends spent writing this book. I'd also like to thank my co-author for making that writing fun and interesting. Special thanks to Norma and Leon Siegel for invaluable feedback on text and illustrations.

LaRiena Ralph
I would like to thank Steve Siegel for the privilege of working on a subject that means so much to me. I'd like to thank Steve, Paul Moberg and Christian Kohler for giving me the opportunity to make so many of the decisions that helped me truly know our patients, their families, and the difficult situations they face every day. I'd also like to thank my friends in the Brain and Behavior Lab at the University of Pennsylvania for being so supportive, working so hard as a team and making it such a pleasurable experience. I'm happy to have been a part of it all. Thank you to Angela Nagele and John Ralph for reading all the drafts and supporting my every decision in life. I have a few special thanks for people unnamed, I appreciate your time, endless support and willingness to share your story—Thank you.

We'd both like to thank our colleagues at Penn and Jones and Bartlett Publishers for help and guidance with this project. Most importantly, we wish to thank the patients and families who provided the perspectives and vignettes that motivated and contributed to this work. We truly appreciate the privilege of having worked with you all.

1 ■ Diagnosing Schizophrenia

The *Diagnostic and Statistical Manual of Mental Disorders* (DSM) is a classification system that forms the most currently accepted clinical standard for diagnosing all psychiatric illness. Each psychiatric disorder is described by a set of diagnostic criteria. The DSM was first published in 1952, and five revisions have been released since that time. The last major revision was in 1994, resulting in the 4th edition, termed DSM-IV. A subsequent minor modification was added in 2000, now referred to as the DSM-IV-TR (text revision). The next major revision, expected to be named DSM-V, is planned for release in 2011. Using DSM-IV guidelines, once a diagnosis is established, the likelihood of a certain outcome is described based on the predictive validity of a constellation of symptoms, or other criteria over time. Each individual's situation over time can change based on circumstances. These dynamic changes are described using five domains, called the multiaxial system. This multiaxial system parses contributing factors into the following:

- Psychiatric diagnosis.
- Personality.
- Medical comorbidity.
- Psychosocial stressors and overall level of function.

Axis I

Axis I describes major psychiatric conditions and associated lifelong conditions that have profound effects on a person's behavior and life course. The following are examples of these disorders:

- Psychiatric disorders: Schizophrenia, bipolar disorder, major depression, generalized anxiety disorder, obsessive compulsive disorder, and so on.
- Developmental disorders: Asperger's, autism, pervasive developmental disorder, and so on.

- Learning disorders: Reading, mathematics, generalized, and so on.

Axis II

Axis II are stable personality traits or disorders that are organized in three clusters, labeled as A through C:

- **Cluster A:** Psychosis-like personality types: Paranoid (suspicious), schizoid (isolative), schizotypal (odd, eccentric).
- **Cluster B:** Depressive personality with patterns of disruptive and sociopathic behaviors:
  - Antisocial: Violent, persistent disregard for others, dishonest.
  - Borderline: Dramatic instability in interpersonal relationships, manipulative, demanding.
  - Histrionic: Excessive need for approval, attention-seeking, dramatic, tend to be flirtatious/seductive in nature.
  - Narcissistic: Overvalued sense of self-worth and entitlement, lack of empathy, often considered self-centered.
- **Cluster C:** Anxious personality types: Avoidant (passive), dependent (needy, clingy), obsessive-compulsive personality (preservative, ritualistic).

Mental retardation is also located on axis II due to the enduring nature of the condition.

Axis III

Axis III describes medical conditions. These are included in the multiaxial system of diagnosis because they may contribute to the patient's overall state of mental health and contribute to the observed clinical picture. Such medical conditions include diabetes, Huntington's disorder, Parkinson's disease, and seizure disorder.

Axis IV

Axis IV includes psychosocial stressors in the patient's life that may contribute to his or her psychological presentation. These are

91–100	Superior functioning in a wide range of activities, life's problems never seem to get out of hand, is sought out by others because of his or her many qualities. No symptoms.
81–90	Absent or minimal symptoms, good functioning in all areas, interested and involved in a wide range of activities, socially effective, generally satisfied with life, no more than everyday problems or concerns.
71–80	If symptoms are present, they are transient and expectable reactions to psychosocial stresses; no more than slight impairment in social, occupational, or school functioning.
61–70	Some mild symptoms OR some difficulty in social, occupational, or school functioning, but generally functioning pretty well, has some meaningful interpersonal relationships.
51–60	Moderate symptoms OR any moderate difficulty in social, occupational, or school functioning.
41–50	Serious symptoms OR any serious impairment in social, occupational, or school functioning.
31–40	Some impairment in reality testing or communication OR major impairment in several areas, such as work or school, family relations, judgment, thinking, or mood.
21–30	Behavior is considerably influenced by delusions or hallucinations OR serious impairment in communications or judgment OR inability to function in all areas.
11–20	Some danger of hurting self or others OR occasionally fails to maintain minimal personal hygiene OR gross impairment in communication.
1–10	Persistent danger of severely hurting self or others OR persistent inability to maintain minimum personal hygiene OR serious suicidal act with clear expectation of death.
0	Not enough information available to provide GAF.

■ **Figure 1.1** **Global Assessment of Function scale.**

Global Assessment of Functioning (GAF) is a scale used in psychiatry to rate the overall level of social, occupational, and psychological functioning of adults. Data from *Diagnostic and Statistical Manual of Mental Disorders*, 2000.

noted as they may contribute to precipitating factors for a psychiatric condition or exacerbate existing conditions. Additionally, these issues provide a context in which the physician can interpret the observed behaviors. Examples of significant stressors include death of a spouse, loss of a job, moving homes, and the birth of a child.

Axis V

Axis V is a Global Assessment of Functioning (GAF) scale that describes a person's overall level of function from 0 (poor function) to 100 (good function). Inpatient hospitalization is generally consistent with a level of 20 or less (Figure 1.1).

Clinical case studies and vignettes will be used throughout the remaining chapters to illustrate various aspects of schizophrenia. Although all cases are based on real stories, some of the demographic and contextual details have been modified to protect the confidentiality of the individuals.

Diagnostic Criteria for Schizophrenia

As with all psychiatric diagnoses, schizophrenia remains a behaviorally defined illness. Diagnostic criteria for schizophrenia according to the *Diagnostic and Statistical Manual of Mental Disorders* (4th edition, text revision—DSM-IV-TR) includes a constellation of positive and negative symptoms lasting longer than 6 months, significant disability, and a lack of other obvious causes (Figure 1.2) (American Psychological Association, 2000).

Positive symptoms are named for the **presence** of behaviors that should not normally exist. These include:

- **Hallucinations**—False sensory experiences that may occur in all modalities.
- **Delusions**—Fixed false beliefs that are inconsistent with the individual's cultural belief.
- **Disorganization**—Including thoughts, speech, and behavior.

Negative symptoms are named for the **lack** of normal behaviors or capabilities that would otherwise be present. These include:

- **Alogia**—Decreased speech.
- **Anhedonia**—The lack of emotion.
- **Asociality**—The lack of normal social interactions or drive.
- **Avolition** or **amotivation**—The lack of desire to do things and lack of action.
- **Affective flattening**—The lack of facial expression and normal body language.

An individual must have at least two positive symptoms or one positive symptom and one negative symptom to meet the so-called **criteria A** for the illness. There are, however, a few symptoms that can fulfill these criteria alone. These include bizarre delusions, defined as beliefs that are not possible (e.g., "an alien living inside my head directing my behavior") as opposed to thoughts that are unlikely albeit possible (e.g., "the police and CIA are tapping my phone and following me around"). The other symptom that can fulfill criteria A alone is a running commentary of voices, which typically consists of an auditory hallucination that announces the individual's thoughts and movements in real time or two or more voices conversing with each other.

The difference between **hallucinations** and **ruminations** is an important distinction that is often overlooked by clinicians. Hallucinations are best defined as true sensory experiences, indistinguishable from the sensation of real external stimuli. For example, many patients deny hallucinations, stating that they have developed extraordinary hearing that enables them to overhear conversations through walls or over great distances. The sensation can then become positive reinforcement for delusions of superior hearing or mind reading, and it can provide content for other delusional beliefs. Alternatively, "thoughts in one's head" that are distinct from true sensory experiences are best regarded as ruminations and should not be ascribed to abnormalities in the perceptual domain.

In addition to the symptomatic criteria, there are requirements for both sufficient duration and disability to justify a diagnosis of schizophrenia. The functional requirement for schizophrenia is designated **criteria B**. To receive a diagnosis of schizophrenia, an individual must display **social or occupational decline** as evident by a marked decline in function with either loss of previous milestones or failure to progress to an expected level. For example, patients may drop out of school, develop inability to work, or become unable to care for their home and family despite previously normal development. To meet criteria for schizophrenia,

---

Criteria A—Positive and Negative Symptoms: At least two of the following must be present

1. Delusions (bizarre delusions alone are sufficient)
2. Disorganization (behavior, speech, or thought process)
3. Hallucinations (a voice commenting or voices conversing is sufficient)
4. Negative symptoms (alogia, anhedonia, asociality, avolition, affective flattening)

Criteria B—Social or Occupational Decline: The person demonstrates a marked decline in function with either loss of previous milestones or failure to progress to expected level. For example, patients may experience dropping out of school, inability to work, or inability to care for home and family despite previously normal development.

Criteria C—Duration: Criteria A and B must be present for at least 6 months. Following treatment, positive symptoms may be diminished or disappear. Negative symptoms and functional decline generally persist during treatment.

■ Figure 1.2   Diagnostic criteria for schizophrenia according to DSM-IV-TR.

the symptoms (criteria A) and disability (criteria B) must also be present for a sufficient duration to rule out less severe or temporary conditions. The duration requirement is called **criteria C** and is operationally defined as a period of at least **6 months**. If the individual is successfully treated with medication, positive symptoms may diminish or disappear during this interval. However, negative symptoms and functional decline generally persist during treatment. The rationale for adding the 6-month duration criterion stems from the observation that other diagnoses or acute causes will become increasingly less likely as time goes by. For example, depressive disorders, medical conditions, or drug abuse will either resolve or become apparent over the course of 6 months of observation. Additionally, complicating factors such as bereavement or other extreme psychosocial stressors will become less contributory.

Types of Schizophrenia

Schizophrenia is a heterogeneous illness with a great deal of variation in both the presentation and severity. In recognition of this variability, four categories have been defined by the relative weight of different symptom clusters—paranoid, catatonic, disorganized, and undifferentiated—as well as a fifth category defined by late-stage illness (residual).

The **paranoid** type is characterized by a relative prominence of delusions and/or severe hallucinations without severe disorganization, catatonia (immobility), or negative symptoms. All domains may be present, but the most severe dimensions in this type of schizophrenia are hallucinations and delusions. The paranoid type is thought to have a good outcome relative to other types. This may reflect a more benign form of illness or unique neurobiology and etiology. Alternatively, it likely reflects the fact that current medications are effective for hallucinations and delusions but do little for catatonia or negative symptoms. Thus, paranoid schizophrenia is a form of the illness that is marked by treatable symptoms and thus may appear more manageable.

The **catatonic** type is a relatively severe form of schizophrenia that is characterized by catalepsy or immobility with waxy flexibility; echolalia or echopraxia (reflexive repetition of words or motions of another person); negativism or resistance to physical or verbal directions; maintenance of a rigid, inappropriate posture; mutism; stereotopies or repetitive purposeless movements; and grimacing. At least two of these behaviors must be present to meet criteria for catatonic schizophrenia. The extent to which catatonic symptoms exist is variable across the course of illness. Unlike other symptoms of schizophrenia, catatonia is often responsive to benzodiazepines (tranquilizers such as Valium or Ativan). However, once the effects of the medication wear off, the catatonia returns until the underlying cause is addressed. Thus it is crucial to recognize that catatonia can be a manifestation of many illnesses. For example, it is difficult to diagnose schizophrenia during the catatonic phase, because catatonia itself can also be a manifestation of depression. If depression is the underlying cause, then electroconvulsive therapy is particularly helpful and often required. The diagnosis of schizophrenia must generally be made during a nonmute/noncatatonic period.

The **disorganized** type of schizophrenia is intermediate in severity and prognosis; it is categorized between the relatively benign paranoid type and the more severe catatonic type. Disorganized schizophrenia is characterized by a prominence of disorganized behavior and speech in the presence of flat or inappropriate affect.

The **undifferentiated** type is diagnosed due to a lack of prominence for any single symptom constellation in the presence of sufficient symptoms to meet the threshold for schizophrenia.

The final category, **residual** type, is orthogonal to the previous groups in that it is marked by the absence of prominent positive symptoms in the presence of negative symptoms and disability. The lack of positive symptoms may result from successful treatment. Thus, residual schizophrenia is defined by the dimensions of schizophrenia that are amenable to current treatment modalities. As noted above, most antipsychotic medications diminish positive symptoms such as hallucinations, delusions, and disorganization. However they are not effective for negative symptoms and do little to restore function (Arango, Buchanan, Kirkpatrick, & Carpenter, 2004). Alternatively, residual schizophrenia may be diagnosed late in the illness because positive symptoms tend to subside over time. Positive symptoms may be seen as analogous to a raging fire during the exacerbations early in the illness but tend to subside later on in life. This observation led to the term *burnt out* schizophrenia, which was occasionally used in the past to relay the clinical observation that the most visible and dramatic symptoms of schizophrenia may fade over time.

There is an additional dimension called **deficit syndrome** that can be added as a modifier to the aforementioned categories based on prominence of negative symptoms (Carpenter, 1994; Carpenter, Heinrichs, & Wagman, 1988; Wagman, Heinrichs, & Carpenter, 1987). Although deficit syndrome is not part of the formal DSM-IV-R scheme, the deficit category is defined as prominent negative symptoms that can not be attributed to depression or medication side effects (Carpenter et al., 1988). Individuals with this constellation of symptoms display relatively isolated lives in the absence of significant motivation, interpersonal contacts, emotional connection, or role functioning. This modifier has been particularly useful since the presence of deficit syndrome has both functional and prognostic significance. Several studies suggest that the presence of deficit syndrome is predictive of poor outcome (Arango et al., 2004; Fenton & McGlashan, 1994; Mayerhoff et al., 1994).

Unfortunately, there is no real guideline to indicate which antipsychotic medications are more or less effective for the different subtypes of schizophrenia. As noted above, benzodiazepines are used as temporary measures in catatonia. No agents are particularly helpful for negative or cognitive problems. Thus, these illness dimensions do not contribute to a rational therapeutic strategy. Clinicians typically choose a medication and dose based on the positive symptoms. For example, if positive symptoms remain, the dose is escalated. Other factors include side effect profiles and personal preference of the physician and patient. If the patient experiences a high degree of motor side effects as the dose is escalated, switching to another agent may be required. These aspects are discussed at greater length in Chapter 6 (Medications).

Non-DSM Signs and Symptoms

Cognitive Deficits

The DSM-IV-R definition captures the most obvious manifestations of schizophrenia, but it does not address other aspects that have emerged as important therapeutic targets and determinants of outcome. For example, schizophrenia is marked by profound cognitive disabilities that leave patients unable to perform many simple tasks or maintain vocational or role-appropriate function (e.g., employment, student, or homemaker) (Green, Kern, & Heaton, 2004; Green & Nuechterlein, 2004; Gur, Ragland, Moberg, Bilker, et al., 2001; Gur, Ragland, Moberg, Turner, et al., 2001). This has become an area of intense research and clinical interest in recent years. Despite earlier claims that new medications had superior effect on cognitive outcome, this assertion has not been substantiated (Siegel et al., 2006). The National Institutes of Health (NIH) and the Food and Drug Administration (FDA) have attempted to address this gap in therapeutic development by sponsoring a consensus panel. This panel, entitled Measurement and Treatment Research to Improve Cognition in Schizophrenia (MATRICS), was created to define cognitive domains, tasks, and targets for future drug development (Geyer & Heinssen, 2005; Green & Nuechterlein, 2004; Marder, Fenton, & Youens, 2004). The MATRICS initiative is intended to provide a framework to standardize criteria for assessing cognitive function and therefore for demonstrating cognitive improvement (Green & Nuechterlein, 2004). However, there is still no clear consensus that the MATRICS battery will be adopted among pharmaceutical companies that may favor faster more automated computerized batteries that offer increased reliability, standardization across clinical sites, and ease of use. Such test batteries are being rapidly developed in a variety of settings with some made freely available (Figure 1.3) (Gur, Ragland, Moberg, Bilker, et al., 2001).

Insight

Although insight is a difficult concept to quantify, many patients with schizophrenia lack the ability to clearly perceive the nature of their situation. That is to say, they lack insight into their illness and how it affects many facets of their lives. Indeed, some experts note that impaired insight is the most prevalent symptom of the disorder, with estimates of impaired insight as high as 95%. Impaired insight is a major source of both interpersonal discord and nonadherence to medication. The following case studies illustrate how poor insight has a devastating effect on patients and their families.

■ Poor Insight—CASE STUDY 1.1

Source: The patient is a 49-year-old male who appears to be his stated age. He is seen in clinical consultation at the request of his lawyer.

History of present illness: The patient is currently seeking reinstatement at a former job at the US Post Office as part of his legal action. However, this evaluation was clinical in nature and not intended as either proof or disproof of disability or fitness for work. The patient was interviewed in the presence of his lawyer and wife at his request. Records were reviewed from previous medical evaluations.

The patient describes the reason for coming as "my lawyer wanted me to." Additionally, he is motivated by his assertion of being inappropriately labeled with a psychiatric condition at 25 years of age and that the label of having a psychiatric condition has adversely affected his life.

Patient states he had a normal childhood, except for a problem with back pain since high school and urinary incontinence "all my life." He states he did well in high school, had lots of friends, and went to college following graduation. At college, he switched majors

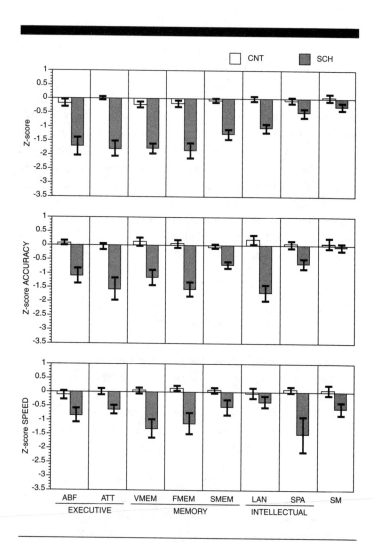

■ Figure 1.3   The neurocognitive profile of patients with schizo-
                phrenia and healthy controls (mean +/- SEM) on the
                traditional battery (top bar) and the computerized
                scan accuracy (middle) and speed (bottom).

three times over the course of 5 years and completed only 3 years of work, leaving without a diploma. He then worked a variety of jobs that culminated in an ultimatum from his mother that he either get a "real job" or join the military. He joined the US Air Force at age 25. After approximately 3 months in the Air Force, he was involved in an automobile accident that resulted in exacerbation of previous back pain. He describes tooth pain at that time and demonstrates how it affected the entire side of his face. His interactions with military medical doctors at that time resulted in psychiatric evaluation and inpatient psychiatric hospitalization lasting 6 months across two facilities with an eventual medical discharge from the service and a diagnosis of schizophrenia. Documentation from that time indicates the patient was disorganized and had multiple somatic complaints that could not be accounted for following appropriate evaluation. Among these were reports that he thought his genitals were "ugly." Patient now states he made up those complaints for various reasons, albeit in the context of currently trying to have the diagnosis of schizophrenia reversed.

Following military service, the patient went to trade school for electronics, but eventually obtained a position at the US Post Office. While at the post office, he had persistent and repeated difficulties with multiple dismissals, all of which he ascribes to the actions of others. For example, the patient believes one supervisor was stalking him and that a group of workers were harassing him because he was too qualified to work in their group. Another time he states his records were left out where they could be seen and his personal life was exposed. He believes the trouble originated from his decision to act as advocate for his wife during a labor dispute early in his position there. He describes sleep disturbances all his life, which he states "are why I can work the graveyard shift." This too has been an object of contention at his previous job.

Medical history: Patient describes urinary incontinence all his life and back pain.

Medications: No psychiatric medications at this time

Social history: He is married with one son age 16, who is currently in high school and without difficulties. Records indicate that the patient's wife has also been diagnosed with either schizophrenia or bipolar disorder in different records. The relevance of his wife's condition pertains to the risk of illness in their son. If both parents have schizophrenia, then there is a 50% chance that their offspring will also be affected. The patient denies ever having a drinking problem but states he had several drinks a day in college and more in the military, which he rationalizes as "normal" for those settings. He does not appear to meet criteria for dependence at any time. There is no history of drug abuse.

Family history: He has two sisters and one brother. He states there is no family history of psychiatric illness. His father died of cardiac illness.

Mental status exam:

Behavior: Patient was cooperative with exam, although there was a clear agenda evident in his answers.

Speech: Normal rate, volume, and rhythm with mild pressure at times during which he spoke over the interviewer and insisted on continuing his responses despite being asked to move to the next topic.

Mood: "Fine" with mostly congruous affect, which became irritable when pressed on issues he did not like. Behavior was mildly antagonistic at times, without any evidence of danger or aggression.

Affect: Full range, irritated but congruent with content of discussion.

Thought process: Tangential, requiring frequent redirection and strained interview from both myself and his lawyer; consistent with mild to moderate thought disorder.

Thought content: Evaluation was compromised by clear agenda to reverse prior diagnoses. However, he adheres to the belief that all of his problems are due to external forces and people and that all of his medical problems are real and simply have not been appropriately diagnosed (cold extremities and genitalia). He denies any thoughts of self-harm or wish to harm others. He appears to lack the capacity for introspection and self-assessment, becoming visibly annoyed when pressed even slightly to consider alternative explanations for his problems.

Perception: He denies present or previous hallucinations.

Insight: Poor, as evidenced by an inability to entertain or discuss possible reasons for his repeated difficulties over the past 30 years.

Judgment: Poor at times, choosing to use sick leave when he needed to miss work but then objecting to the innuendo that he was sick.

Assessment: Patient is a 49-year-old man with a 30-year history of difficulties with interpersonal relations, repeated difficulties at work, and at times multiple somatic complaints for which no medical cause could be identified. His presentation is strongly colored by his desire to not have a psychiatric illness and his request to be vindicated from his perception of mistreatment at the post office. He exhibits a mildly aggressive and inappropriate posture during the interview, which may be due to suspicion and irritation at seeing yet another doctor. He needs frequent redirection to stay on topic and becomes irritated at the slightest suggestion of his complaints resulting from either psychiatric illness or his own interpersonal style. He shows poor insight regarding the persistent nature of his problems, the role his own actions and decisions have played in his life, and the possibility that he does in fact suffer from a psychiatric condition. The patient has received the diagnosis of schizophrenia at times, and this has been rebutted at other times. As such it requires careful scrutiny in the context of available records and current presentation. In favor of the diagnosis, he displays a persistent pattern of impaired function characterized by early ambivalence during college and followed by repeated difficulties in a variety of work settings. Additionally, he has multiple somatic complaints that are not consistent with his medical examinations, including incontinence, pain, and coldness. Although he now explains he "made it up," he apparently reported that his penis was malformed during his time in the military. Indeed, he inquired point blank, "What delusions would I have?" to which I responded "Somatic delusion." This is consistent with the findings of earlier examinations that were not available prior to exam. However, even if these complaints are somatic delusions, they are mild and not out of the realm of possibility. Arguing against the diagnosis, the patient has remained married, attempts to work despite his perceived slights, and thus lacks significant negative symptoms. Given the lack of hallucinations, criteria for schizophrenia would rest on thought disorder (mild), somatic delusions (mild), with poor social and occupational function for greater than 6 months without other obvious causes. Indeed this is far from clear. However, no other diagnosis seems more appropriate given the gestalt of his history. His assertion that everything has resulted from forces outside himself is unrealistic given the extent, persistence, and breadth of his problems across multiple settings since his attempt to complete college.

Differential diagnosis includes:

Axis I: Schizophrenia spectrum—Mild manifestations of the full-blown syndrome versus bipolar disorder, type II (see Chapter 2, Differential Diagnosis: Psychiatric Causes), with periods of extreme irritability and psychotic episodes and symptoms, which could also explain much of the patient's difficulty. Such a diagnosis would account for periods of extreme anxiety and irritability with overvalued ideas and interpersonal difficulties, poor sleep, poor insight, and periods of mild psychosis.

Axis II: Consistent with cluster A disorders, specifically paranoid and schizotypal forms. However, this diagnosis can not coexist with a primary axis I psychotic disorder. Thus, an alternate diagnosis to schizophrenia is bipolar II with cluster A personality disorder.

Axis III: Urinary incontinence and back pain.

Axis IV: His job and perception of being mistreated are his primary stressors.

Axis V: 60–70.

Recommendations: It is not likely that this patient could effectively reintegrate into any work setting in the absence of pharmacological treatment. Given the diagnostic uncertainty between schizophrenia spectrum and bipolar II, a low-dose antipsychotic such as Zyprexa or risperidone would be most appropriate (see Chapter 6, Medications). Alternatively, valproate or lithium would be reasonable first-line efforts if this was preferable to the patient and his treating psychiatrist.

Addendum: Later visits revealed that the patient's wife also had schizophrenia. Both parents lacked insight and were resistant to the idea that their teenage son was at high risk (see Chapter 4, Etiology). They were lost to follow-up.

■ **Poor Insight Leading to Family Discord**—CASE STUDY 1.2
Source: Patient and her son during interview.

History of present illness: Patient is a 46-year-old female seen at the behest of her son. She states there is a rift between her and her 30-year-old son, which she believes is due to the influence of her family, her daughter-in-law, and her daughter-in-law's family. The patient states that everything was fine until she moved south from New York to South Carolina. While there, she states she became involved with a man who has stalked her and continues to influence her life. Despite having moved back north, she changed her phone number several times, using only post office boxes, to avoid revealing her address. She believes this man has tapped her phone, bugged her car, and spread rumors about her on the Internet and radio. She's had her car checked for microphones by mechanics and requested protection from police. She believes that on a recent trip to Connecticut, he influenced the band to play, "Going to Carolina" as a signal, and that her brother was "in on it" because he looked at her when the song started, further signifying that he knew what it meant. Additionally, she states that everyone in her town talks about her, that her extended family is involved and plotting against her, and that they have influenced her son to be against her as well. She states most of her life has been unpleasant, and that "bad luck" accounts for her string of jobs—she is constantly losing or walking out on her employment due to her beliefs that either some person is sexually harassing her or accusing her of things she did not do. She recently disappeared for several months, during which time she stayed with friends and family in Virginia.

She had her son at age 16, while married. She divorced 3–4 years later after being separated for 2 years. She then raised her son as a single mother. She states that she has the ability to read people's mind by reading their lips, and has premonitions of events that date back over 20 years. For example, she states she had a dream that her son would drown when he was 9, and the next day he fell in a pool. When asked if it might be the case that she was simply concerned about taking him to a pool, knowing that he could not swim, she stated that "it was a premonition." Similarly, she states that she had a dream that something terrible would happen to him when he was 4, and he cut his finger the next day. Additionally, she states she is able to take pain from him; for example, when he was younger, she would take his stomachache, and "have it for him." She currently complains of abdominal pain, for which her gastroenterologist prescribes Zoloft after all medical workup failed to relieve the pain. She also complains of lethargy and depressed mood at times. She adds that people have been in her house, and people from her former job entered her house to delete files from her computer. She currently works as an administrative assistant and sells real estate on weekends. She denies periods of elevated mood, although she does describe irritability. She cries at times but does not ever think of harming herself. She is guarded and suspicious, not revealing her Social Security number on intake forms. She also asked for copies of all documents and refused to answer family history questions but would not go into detail as to why.

She believes she gives off an odor, which her son believes is an olfactory hallucination. He states that it started as simple concern about bad breath, then became underarm odor complaints—now she believes her breath wreaks of urine. She states the odor is real, and that others are simply being polite when they deny it. No odor was detected at the interview.

Past medical history: GI upset, negative workup, treated with Zoloft by her gastroenterologist, also reports a lump under her arm, which is being followed by surgeon. Previously took St. John's wort "prophylactically" and takes candied ginger for her stomach, having recently discontinued "natural" digestive enzymes at the request of her gastroenterologist.

Social history: Patient is single, working as an administrative assistant. She formerly worked at similar jobs as well as a waitress. No drug use. Married at 16, divorced at 20. She has been in several long-term and shorter relationships. Not currently involved with anyone.

Medications: Zoloft 25 mg per day, candied ginger from health food store.

Mental status exam:

Behavior: Pleasant and guarded initially, later more cooperative as interview progressed.

Speech: Normal volume and rate.

Mood: Upset over relationship with son.

Affect: Full range.

Thought process: Linear.

Thought content: No suicidal or homicidal thoughts. Delusions of reference and persecution as well as somatic delusions present, "I think something is wrong, even though they never find anything."

Perception: Olfactory hallucinations suspected, denies auditory or visual disturbances.

Insight: Poor: "I know it's all real. This can't be in my head."

Judgment: Poor: "If you can't make them stop, then you can't do anything for me."

Assessment: 46-year-old woman with psychosis. Differential diagnosis includes schizophrenia, as evidenced by greater than 7-year history of delusion, poor function, and suggestion of olfactory hallucinations. Bipolar disorder, with episodes of hypomania is also possible. However, the presence of frank psychosis is inconsistent with bipolar type II.

Recommendations: Patient informed that treatment with antipsychotic medication is definitely indicated and should be pursued. She refuses. Despite the patient's initial refusal to return for treatment, she was given a prescription for risperidone, 1 mg at bedtime, with the hope that she would change her mind and pursue care. She was strongly advised to consider treatment.

Addendum: The patient's psychosis continued, leading to increasing discord between her and her son's family. Eventually, she was not able to interact with her grandchildren secondary to concerns that her psychotic content might lead her to interact poorly with them and/or run away with them. Despite this devastating consequence of her refusal to comply with care, she persisted in believing that her delusions were real. This case demonstrates the strength with which many patients adhere to their beliefs, even when doing so causes such a devastating outcome.

Sensory and Motor Abnormalities

Sensory Deficits of Schizophrenia

While most studies focus on higher cognitive processes, recent data indicate that patients with schizophrenia have deficits in basic processing of sensory stimuli. These deficits have been best studied in the auditory modality but are present across all senses. For example, patients have profound difficulty with the sense of smell, both in terms of sensitivity and the ability to assign hedonic valance (e.g., pleasant versus unpleasant). Electroencephalography (EEG) has been widely used to study sensory-processing deficits in schizophrenia. Specifically, EEG responses to auditory stimuli are recorded and averaged to yield event-related potentials (ERPs). Human ERPs are characterized by a positive voltage deflection occurring approximately 50 milliseconds (ms) after the stimulus (P50) and a negative voltage deflection occurring 100 ms after the stimulus (N100). Although not discussed as often as their preceding components in the context of gating or habituation, the P200 and P300 are positive deflections occurring 200 and 300 ms poststimulus, respectively. In the paired click paradigm, component amplitudes elicited by the first stimulus (S1) are normally greater than equivalent potentials elicited by a second stimulus (S2), delivered, generally, 500 ms later. However, several studies suggested that schizophrenic individuals exhibit similar response amplitudes to both stimuli, yielding a lower ratio between them (Adler et al., 1982; Boutros, Zouridakis, & Overall, 1991). This gating deficit may result from a decreased response to the first stimulus and/or a failure to inhibit the second stimulus.

Motor Manifestations of Schizophrenia

Although antipsychotic medication treatment can cause motor impairments such as stiffness (Chapter 6, Medications), schizophrenia itself can include abnormalities in coordination and movement (Kopala, 1996). These problems can be subtle, requiring a neurological exam to reveal, or they can be grossly apparent as in the form of tardive dyskinesia (TD) (Fenton, Wyatt, & McGlashan, 1994). Tardive dyskinesia is a late-onset, age-dependent emergence of abnormal movements (Fenton, Blyler, Wyatt, & McGlashan, 1997). The incidence of TD increases with age, such that approximately 40% of schizophrenia patients will exhibit TD by 60 years of age (Fenton, 2000). One of the greatest misconceptions in psychiatry today is that antipsychotic medications cause TD. However, there is substantial evidence that TD is actually part of the illness rather than a manifestation of treatment. This evidence includes the following:

- Tardive dyskinesia in schizophrenia was described in the late 1800s, over 50 years prior to the discovery of the first antipsychotic medication.
- Approximately 40% of schizophrenia patients develop TD in the absence of treatment (Fenton, 2000). This has been demonstrated both by observing its incidence in patients that refuse treatment and in countries that do not have access to medication.

There is evidence that treatment may alter the extent and incidence of TD risk; however, these studies must always be interpreted on the background of age-emergent expression of TD as a normal part of schizophrenia.

Emotional Recognition

Deficits in emotional expression, or flat affect, have been a well-recognized aspect of schizophrenia for many years. More recently, there has been wider recognition that individuals with schizophrenia also have difficulties in recognizing emotions of other people. For example, patients are less able to accurately identify the emotion being portrayed by a facial expression in a photograph. Similarly, they are less able to accurately rate the strength of emotion. For example, a picture of a very angry face may be interpreted by schizophrenia patients as neutral or only mildly annoyed. Conversely, a neutral expression may be misread as angry. Since a great deal of communication between people involves such nonverbal cues as facial expression and body language, this deficit leaves many patients unable to accurately read the messages being portrayed by people around them. The inaccurate interpretation of nonverbal cues may contribute to psychotic symptoms if there is the inappropriate perception that someone is angry. Alternatively, patients may suffer from social isolation, to some extent, because of their inadequate ability to communicate through nonverbal cues and therefore participate in the full breath of conversation. As such, this basic inability to interpret emotional meaning can have significant symptomatic impact.

Progression to Onset

Given all of these severe and dramatic manifestations of schizophrenia, one might assume that diagnosis would occur rapidly following onset of difficulties. However, it is generally accepted that the average lag from onset of illness to first medical attention is 2–3 years. There are a number of factors that contribute to this delay. First, early symptoms are generally mild and fall in a continuum of normal, albeit suboptimal behaviors. For example, negative symptoms may begin with quitting social activities at school—a patient that formerly was engaged in clubs or sports may be seen as focusing on school work or maturing. However, this can then progress to further isolation from friends and poor attendance in school that can be interpreted as poor work ethic or teenage angst and uncertainty. Similarly, early signs of positive symptoms may be seen as "a bad situation" in which the family believes that people at school or work really are talking about their child or are being "cliquey" and mean. The following example was written by a young woman with schizophrenia to provide her personal perspective on how her illness unfolded at onset and is illustrative of this typical progression.

> Go to college, meet people, have fun, learn—get a job. This is the typical/normal path most college graduates follow. I just did not know it. I thought there were more options and paths to follow until you got the job that you wanted and were suitable for. As I look at some of my family and friends, I realize that the first choice (school to job) may have not only been a more typical path, but also may have been a better, saner choice. I did not have a path even though I graduated with honors. Instead, I went abroad, took temporary jobs, traveled, went to AmeriCorps—trying to avoid the inevitability of schizophrenia.

Right after college, I worked abroad in England for 6 months. I was on a student/work visa and worked an administrative job in a marketing department. So, in a way, I actually followed the school–job path. I just did it in a different country. For the most part, I was really happy to be there and make new friends and experience a new culture. Despite this, though, I started to feel the early symptoms of schizophrenia. I started to feel like I was being given messages through the media, mainly magazines and a band and musician. At first, it was kind of fun to feel like this was happening. It would only occur (to me) later on, to be a box that I could not escape from.

After London, I came home and did a lot temporary jobs, never really committing myself to any of them. Instead, I traveled to California and New York a lot. When I finally was bored with this, I looked for a full-time, permanent job. Unfortunately, I was not able to get any of the jobs I applied for. As far as my psychosis went, I was getting worse. I started to think that my house was bugged and that the rock band was trying to contact me. I also started to believe that there were messages encoded in my conversations with others.

After I was over this chase that I created, I wanted to escape it and so, since I did not get a job, I looked into volunteering at AmeriCorps. After applying to several different programs, I got a volunteer position in Baltimore. That is when I became psychotic. It was horrifying. I moved into a house with three other people, who I thought were reading my diaries, putting things in my food, and bugging my room. As for the job, I was completely shy, scared, and unsuitable. After I felt too unsafe in the house, I moved to an apartment, where I was doing well for a little bit. Then, things returned to being crazy. I thought that my apartment was bugged and that everyone I worked with was out to get me, invading my privacy, and making me crazy.

After AmeriCorps, I returned home, where my small psychosis turned into a large psychosis. Soon, everything seemed related to me. I thought the media was trying to contact me, that rock stars were driving in my town and trying to contact me, and that I was writing to them. I think now that I look at my choices in retrospect, I can see how it led to my diagnosis of schizophrenia. But, instead of thinking of it as failure in choices, I see it as being a progression of events on the path to schizophrenia.

The following record is from the physician notes regarding this person's initial evaluation.

New-Onset Schizophrenia—CASE STUDY 1.3

Source: Patient and both parents.

History of present illness: Patient is a 25-year-old female who was brought to the ER approximately 1 month after she attacked her father in a restaurant. She was evaluated and released from ER at that time.

The patient describes herself as having always been shy, with average grades in high school, earning a B average. She then went to college where she majored in psychology and obtained a GPA of 3.8. After college, she moved to England where, according to her parents, she thrived and functioned independently for 6 months. Upon returning to the United States, she worked at temp agencies in several jobs. She later joined the AmeriCorps and moved from rural Pennsylvania to urban Maryland.

She states that difficulties began while working at AmeriCorps in Maryland. At that time she believed that one of her housemates climbed through her window from outside and frightened her. She denies any physical contact or assault, but states she left the house that night and never returned. During the following month, she began to believe that people at work knew her business and that they were hanging around her apartment. She states someone mentioned they had seen a person in a blue coat. She associated this with blue coats worn at work. She also complains that someone came into her apartment and "switched the yogurt." She returned to live with her parents in the summer of 1998 "due to the stress" of the above events. She states that the first month was fine, then there was increasing tension between her and her parents. She became increasingly violent with episodes of breaking glasses, punching a hole in a wall, and kicking a hole in a bathtub tile. She was hospitalized on a voluntary admission after she wandered out of the house for 2 hours in a storm. She states she had gone to a restaurant instead of wandering for 2 hours as her parents contended. Discharge diagnosis was depression, without psychotic features according to the patient. During this period she also left home one time and did not return for 2 days, during which her parents had her movements tracked by credit card use. She was hospitalized again on an involuntary commitment that was extended by the court for 2 weeks of inpatient treatment with court-mandated aftercare and medication. The patient had an altercation with her parents at that time and threw keys at her father after accusing them of stealing her keys. Discharge diagnosis was schizophrenia. She then engaged in treatment with her psychiatrist who began treating her with risperidone, 4 mg per day, initiated in the hospital. Her psychiatrist made the preliminary diagnosis of post-traumatic stress syndrome (PTSD). The patient's mother added they were counting her pills periodically and, at that time, she would miss approximately one third of the days. Her mother stated that all family members were extremely concerned, as they felt she had deteriorated so much. Her mother also described episodes of frequent outbursts with cursing.

Her psychiatrist reports that when he first met the patient she was guarded and stated that she could not speak because "he" was listening, referring to a rock star who she believed was monitoring her at all times. She also reported an evil force that affected her and that her parents were being influenced. She stated that she had flashback experiences "reliving" the episode when her housemate broke into her room and a possible encounter at another time. Her psychiatrist reports that the patient became increasingly vague and refused medications at that time. She also displayed giggling as well as emotional outbursts.

Past medical history: No known illnesses. Patient tested "high normal" for Antinuclear Antibody (ANA) titler.

Family history: Family history of alcoholism, depression, and a "nervous breakdown" with repeated hospitalizations, and "anxiety disorder" as well as lupus.

Social history: Presently living with her family and unemployed; no past or present history of drug or alcohol use.

Medications: Risperidone, 4 mg at bedtime. The patient discontinued taking her medication once the court mandate expired.

Mental status exam:

Appearance: Mildly disheveled with loose-fitting clothing, inappropriate to situation.

Behavior: Partially cooperative with silly affect at times laughing inappropriately.

Speech: Normal.

Mood: "OK."

Affect: Intermittently inappropriate laughter.

Thought process: Linear and logical.

Thought content: Without delusional, suicidal, or homicidal ideation; no evidence of referential thinking or persecutory ideas.

Perception: No perceptual abnormalities.

Insight: Very poor: "There is no problem."

Judgment: Poor: e.g., She stood up in a restaurant and yelled, "I'll kill the fucking bastards," then wanted to continue eating there and could not understand why they had to leave.

Assessment: 24-year-old female with symptoms consistent with schizophreniform illness of approximately 1 year duration including social and occupational decline, social withdrawal, disorganization, inappropriate affect, periods of delusions of a bizarre nature, as well as referential and persecutory ideation. Therefore, her symptoms are most consistent with a diagnosis of schizophrenia—paranoid vs. disorganized subtype (see page 7 regarding types of schizophrenia).

As noted in the previous account, the progression to onset of schizophrenia often has elements of depression (sadness), mania (irritability or excitement), anxiety (nervousness), or confusion (overwhelmed), as well as changes in interests and social interactions. These features are not specific to any one diagnosis, or even necessarily indicative of illness. In addition, the most prominent signs and symptoms within an individual may shift over time, challenging diagnostic categories and stability. However, a careful and systematic assessment of the life course can often help delineate one diagnosis from another. The following chapter uses a series of case reports to illustrate how the constellation of symptoms and progression over time coalesce to indicate a specific diagnosis.

2 ■ Differential Diagnosis: Psychiatric Conditions to Distinguish from Schizophrenia

It is important to note that isolated positive and negative symptoms that occur in other medical and psychiatric disorders may overlap with the presentation of schizophrenia. Although the cross-sectional appearance of different conditions may be similar, their long-term prognosis and long-term treatments differ significantly from that of schizophrenia. Alternatively, the acute treatment of hallucinations and delusions from any cause usually involves the same classes of medication.

Psychiatric Disorders to Distinguish from Schizophrenia

The following is a series of cases illustrating both the overlapping and distinguishing features one must consider when diagnosing schizophrenia. Each case illustrates key features of overlap and distinguishing characteristics between diagnoses.

Schizophrenia vs. Depression and Seizure Disorder— Case Study 2.1

Sources: Patient self-report and review of records.

History of present illness: Patient is a 24-year-old female referred for consultation by her primary psychiatrist with a 6-month history of increased difficulties with her mood, thinking, and behavior. She has a history of epileptic seizures, petit and grand mal types, which were treated for approximately 2 years prior to the current series of events. Her last tonic-clonic (grand mal) seizure was approximately 1.5 years prior, and she notes she may have had an absence seizure (petit) a few weeks ago but is not certain.

Following graduation from a highly competitive college, the patient took a corporate position in finance at a major international bank, with increasing levels of advancement over the 2 years following college. She notes she left that position in another city 6 months ago due to a constellation of factors including concerns over her ability to meet the increasing workload, a difficult breakup of a relationship, and unresolved grief over the death of her father years earlier. At that time, she had been in a relationship with a new boyfriend for 3 months. She then moved back to her family home. Following several months in a long-distance relationship, she joined her boyfriend for a trip abroad to visit his family. Within 1 week of arriving, their relationship deteriorated from a "stormy" baseline to the point where she accused him of not being who he said he was and of working for her old boyfriend as part of a plot to harm her in retribution for the breakup. There was also evidence of referential delusions, thinking other people with the same name as her boyfriend were somehow related to him, or actually were him (e.g., if someone was mentioned that had the same name she inferred it to be her ex). She also described an episode in a store in which she believed a customer and salesperson became involved in a plot against her based on comments they made.

In this context, her boyfriend contacted the patient's family and brought her to the local hospital. She was sedated and repatriated to the United States, where her brother escorted her to a hospital. At that hospital, she was initially seen by neurology and then discharged to outpatient psychiatric services. All neurological tests (MRI, CT, EEG, serology, and hematology labs) were within normal limits. Upon completing 1 month of intensive outpatient psychiatric treatment, she moved back in with her boyfriend. While there, she became psychotic again, this time being admitted to inpatient psychiatric services in another city for 1 month. During this period, she describes suicidality, crying, frank delusions as noted above, and periods of catatonia. She was treated with lorazepam, risperidone, and her seizure medication was changed, apparently due to concern that her original medication might contribute to psychosis. She states her symptoms slowly resolved to the point that she was discharged with reduced severity including occasional crying.

She disclosed that she asked her boyfriend to hide all sharp objects after her discharge due to concern she would use them to harm herself. She states he asked her to get a knife one time, which her family thought was inappropriate (by her report). Of note, the episode had a slight "axis II-like quality" in that she placed the locus of control onto another individual in a dramatic way that would make him appear culpable for her own maladaptive behaviors (self-harm). This description led me to ask if she had ever cut herself, to which she reported "thinking about it" and went on to mention having held a knife above her wrist once.

She has remained on the regimen of valproate, risperidone, and lorazapam for the past 2 months. All but occasional crying and sadness related to her current relationship has resolved. No signs of psychosis are currently endorsed.

Past medical history: History of both petit and grand mal seizures. No other medical problems.

Past psychiatric history: She notes she had low self-esteem related to "feeling broken" due to her seizure disorder. She describes some angst during college, for which she received counseling. She also notes a history of stormy relationships with men dating back to high school. She states she had a few periods of decreased sleep (3–4 hr/night for a single night) while in college, denies periods of excessive spending, but admits to some risky sexual behavior following college including unprotected sex with several "one-night stands." She has been tested for HIV and other STDs multiple times and reports being negative for all. She also describes a single episode when she considered but did not follow through with cutting herself. Her ability to readily take responsibility for these decisions argues against either axis I or II etiology for their occurrence.

Social history: She has never used any illicit drugs, does drink *alcohol occasio*nally, has had several relationships with men, and is currently in a strained relationship. She mentioned her surprise that he stayed with her despite her recent events.

Family history: No known history of mental illness.

Mental status exam:

Appearance: She presents as a well-dressed, decently organized woman appearing her age.

Behavior: Appropriate, pleasant demeanor interactive with fully preserved interpersonal skills.

Speech: Normal amount, speed, and volume with normal response latency.

Mood: Is described as "good," although she notes occasional periods of sadness and rare crying.

Affect: Appropriate to the content with full range.

Thought process: Logical and linear.

Thought content: Denies any current delusions, but notes that she had previous periods with both paranoid and referential delusions.

Perception: Denies current or past hallucinations.

Insight: Good. She is aware that her previous behavior was unusual and not rational, and also states she will continue medication.

Judgment: Good. She plans to remain on medication and has returned to her family home while recuperating.

Cognition: Very bright, thoughtful responses to all issues, no signs of difficulty with memory, executive function, or abstraction.

Assessment: The patient is a 24-year-old woman with long history of mild to moderate mood disturbances that escalated and evolved into frank psychosis 6 months ago. The subsequent 6 months have been marked by three inpatient hospitalizations for delusions, suicidality, and catatonia. Her premorbid history has several behavioral elements that do not rise to the level of pathology but either contribute to or complicate diagnosis. These include protracted dysthymia (sadness), periods of reduced sleep, and some risky behaviors that could be interpreted as hypomania. Alternatively, she is a bright, attractive woman who had the opportunity for multiple sexual/romantic relationships and social activities that now take on a retrospective pathological character in the context of current events. Similarly, she describes "stormy" relationships, depressed mood, strained interactions with her family, one episode of thinking about cutting herself, and holding a sharp instrument to her wrist that also take on a retrospective flavor of borderline personality-like behaviors (see Chapter 1, axis II, cluster B for further details). However, these too fail to reach threshold for a true personality disorder given her other interpersonal successes.

Her psychotic episode did occur in the context of treatment with her initial antiseizure medication, which is noted to cause psychosis on rare occasions. The observation that she was not psychotic on this medication for 2 previous years reduces (but does not absolutely rule out) the likelihood that it contributed to her psychiatric symptoms. Her psychosis has resolved since removal of that agent, albeit also in the context of treatment with the antipsychotic medication risperidone. Thus, one cannot disentangle the opposing hypotheses that she either had a medication-induced psychotic episode or a primary psychotic break caused by either a mood disorder or schizophrenia in the context of an unrelated seizure treatment.

Recommendations: The most conservative and appropriate plan of care is to continue all current treatments for a period of 3 months to establish a clear resumption of normalcy. In 3 months, she could reduce lorazepam as tolerated since this was likely initiated to treat the catatonia rather than any underlying cause. Following 6 months with no delusions, outbursts, catatonia, or inpatient hospital, she could slowly reduce the risperidone under the supervision of both a psychiatrist and her family. To do so, I suggest reducing by 0.5 mg every 2 months. If she successfully discontinues risperidone without resumption of psychosis, it will likely have been the seizure medication or bipolar disorder. In that event, she should still continue the valproate for seizures. It remains possible that all of her symptoms were the result of a major depressive episode with psychosis and catatonia. The content of her psychosis argues against that. If, however, her depressed mood returns and is not responsive to therapy, an antidepressant could be explored. However, it is not indicated presently and may complicate more than it clarifies.

Schizophrenia vs. Bipolar Disorder and Alcohol Abuse — CASE STUDY 2.2

Source: Patient, records, and family report.

History of present illness: The patient is a 28-year-old single, white male who carries a diagnosis of bipolar disorder since the age of 26. His father, who met the evaluator during his participation in a family support group, set up the appointment. The patient was seen alone, and requested that I not speak with his parents or his current psychiatrist. He did however agree to allow me to share this record with his primary care physician.

He states that he has had periods of depressed mood going back to his early teens, when he reports he slit his wrists in front of his father. He adds that he is angry with his father for not having taken action then to engage him in psychiatric care at that time. He also reports episodes of "mania," which he describes as periods lasting days or weeks of irritability, aggression, increased/indiscriminant sexual activity at times without condoms, and sleep disturbance. He states he always has poor sleep and therefore has medicated himself with sleeping pills or alcohol to sleep. Therefore, he cannot comment on periods of sleeplessness that are uncomplicated by concurrent alcohol and/or medication. His most recent exacerbation occurred in the context of taking "amino acids" of a nonpharmaceutical source, which he states had "amphetamine" in it. During that period he also described "mania," including spending money on things he didn't need. Although he acknowledges that he has used alcohol in excess on occasion, uses it to relax, and has been involved in altercations while intoxicated, he does not believe alcohol is his primary problem nor one that needs to be addressed with a treatment program. He states his current psychiatrist told him he requires an alcohol cessation program. He adds that his psychiatrist indicated they could not continue to work together if he did not agree to alcohol treatment but then continued his care anyway. Rather than appreciating this as an effort to help him, which is complicated by his own self-destructive behavior, the patient believes his physician only sees him "for the $20 I pay him." He is also angry that his psychiatrist, "could not remember" all the details regarding his various medications and doses.

The patient states he felt like a zombie on a higher dose of lithium, albeit notes that he was also taking an antidepressant and was "depressed" at the time. He distinguishes the feeling from sedation or fatigue, noting it was more characterized by emotional withdrawal.

Medication: His present medications include quetiapine (prescribed 400 mg hs, taking 200 mg) for sleep; lithium (prescribed 450 mg bid, taking 450 mg bid) for bipolar D/O, clonazepam (prescribed 0.5 mg hs, not taking it) for sleep, trazadone (prescribed 100 mg hs prn, not using it) for sleep; Tylenol PM (over-the-counter medication, takes it nightly) for sleep. No lithium level was available at the time of interview.

Medical history: No other illnesses.

Social history: The patient was working full time in a responsible municipal job, although he does have conflicts there resulting in a grievance in which he is claiming discrimination due to his illness. He is also actively dating and has had monogamous relationships in the past. He has several friends with whom he drinks and socializes. He completed college with a degree in communications. He lives with his parents.

Psychiatric history: He has been admitted to a psychiatric hospital previously for affective and behavioral difficulties and required medical leave of absence during his previous psychiatric exacerbation. He was treated at a psychiatric program as a child (at 5 years of age) for behavioral problems. He states the psychiatrist "only played games and talked, indicating that the patient has not developed an understanding of the approach and subsequent benefit that resulted from therapy." He later went on to complete elementary, middle, and high school without further need of intervention.

Mental status exam:

Speech and behavior: Appropriate with normal rate, volume, and prosody.

Mood: Demoralized and angry, with a strong sense that he has been wronged by other people's actions or inactions.

Affect: Full and congruent with mood.

Thought process: Linear and logical in flow.

Thought content: No active suicidal or homicidal thoughts, although he makes provocative comments at times including declining liver function tests "since I don't care if I have a liver problem or not." He displayed a possible presence of delusions of persecution, which may alternatively be a personality style of blaming others for events that are either a direct result of his actions (drinking and arguments) or due to uncontrollable events (illness and occasional conflicts during adolescence).

Perception: There was no evidence of perceptual abnormalities.

Insight: Is poor to moderate as evidenced by an unwillingness to simply stop drinking in the service of clarifying the role of alcohol in his difficulties and inability to think critically about other people's actions and motivation. This is particularly true toward his parents and their efforts to get help for him.

Judgment: Moderate, as evidenced by decisions to take some of his medication and yet continue some maladaptive behaviors despite recognition of their impact.

Assessment: The patient is a 28-year-old single male with bipolar disorder, alcohol abuse, and an argumentative style of interpersonal interactions. He shows some insight into his illness as evidenced by his willingness to see me and take some medication.

However, his anger toward his parents and inability to see things from another perspective and empathize hinders his progress. He also has an unhealthy dependence on daily Tylenol PM. The lack of hallucinations, disorganization, or prominent negative symptoms and his ability to work and express emotion are all less consistent with schizophrenia.

Recommendations: Increase lithium to 450 mg AM and 900 mg PM, checking lithium level after 1 week and titrating up to a dose that yields a serum level of 1.0–1.2. Discontinue Tylenol PM, using trazadone as needed until full effect of lithium is achieved (good sleep, decreased anger/irritability, decreased persecutory ideas). Discontinue clonazepam prescriptions, as he has a problem with alcohol and should avoid other substances that can lead to physical dependence. Discontinue quetiapine, as it is unlikely to be contributing anything beyond a sleep aid. Given lithium use and heavy Tylenol use/abuse, he should have renal and liver function tests. Given periods of indiscriminant-unprotected sex, he should have HIV/hepatitis tests.

If lithium at an appropriate dose fails, he should move to clozapine, starting at 25 mg/day and increasing by 25 mg twice per week until approximately 500 mg per day divided approximately 100 AM/400 PM. At that point, clozapine levels should be checked and titrated until a full treatment effect is achieved with an anticipated serum level of about 500 but no more than 1000.

Schizophrenia vs. Type I Bipolar Disorder—CASE STUDY 2.3

Source: Patient interview.

History of present illness: The patient is a 45-year-old white male who describes onset of symptoms at 17 years of age. He states his diagnoses have included both "manic depression" and schizoaffective disorder. He used marijuana and beer heavily from 13 to 21 years of age and has been completely clean for 24 years. He has had numerous inpatient psychiatric hospitalizations, which he describes as, "too many to go into detail." Before elaborating on his first break, he described his childhood as difficult and tormented by both substance abuse and mental illness in the family. He states he had terrible nightmares throughout childhood, preceding illness.

He describes the first episode as prompted by one of his friends murdering his girlfriend (the friend's, not the patient's). The patient states the event devastated his high school at the time. He became depressed, fearful, isolative, and thought that both the friend who had committed murder and the victim's family would come after him. He stayed in his room and was eventually hospitalized. Since that time he states he has had periods of mania as well as periods of depression, either of which can then incorporate hallucinations and paranoid delusions. However, he believes that he does not experience these symptoms when his mood is "in the middle." He states none of the "old medications" helped him including lithium, haloperidol, trifluoperazine—"all of them"—but that his current regimen (Clozaril, valproate, and Paxil) have kept him well and out of hospital.

He states his hallucinations are not in fact hallucinations, but rather are "clairaudition" and "clairvoyance." However, he does not use the latter term by its usual definition. He has an elaborate theory that normally, stimuli come from outside the physical body, come to the sensory organs, and are turned into electrical energy in the brain. However, he states the reverse can be true, and electrical energy in the brain can go back out the other way, be turned into sound or visual stimuli, which he then experiences as real, albeit they originated within his brain. He adds that this belief system is common to a group of about 20–30 people he meets with weekly in the city. His group believes that there is an "astral body and astral brain" that are made of electricity and magnetism and are responsible for the "inner senses." His mood is normal during the current period during which he rigidly adheres to these ideas.

Family history: Paternal alcoholism and tranquilizer abuse as well as "ADD and bipolar disorder" (not clear if this is his retrospective impression or bona fide diagnoses), his grandmother was institutionalized for schizophrenia, and his grandfather committed suicide.

Medical history: Obesity.

Medications:

Current medication—Clozaril 400 mg, valproate, and Paxil.

Past medications—Haloperidol, trifluoperazine, thorazine, and "all of them."

Social history: He is active in multiple support groups for both addiction and mental illness. He has multiple friends. No active drug or alcohol use for 24 years. He lives independently.

Mental status exam:

Behavior: Pleasant and cooperative.

Speech: Normal volume and rate of speech. He is articulate and engaging with good eye contact. On three occasions he turned his head to the right in a deliberate manner. When asked why, he went into a long elaboration that "No one is perfect, and he would try to maintain better eye contact."

Mood: Good.

Affect: Bright.

Thought process: Tangential and verbose. Answers to simple questions become very elaborate and require 5 minutes rather than a few seconds.

Thought content: Remarkable for odd beliefs about the astral body and astral brain, albeit these may be common to an organized group more akin to cult beliefs than psychosis. No suicidal or homicidal thought.

Perception: He describes auditory and visual hallucinations, limiting them to periods of mood disturbance. He describes these experiences as real sensory experiences that are "so real they can not be imaginary."

Insight and judgment: Good: "The medicines have side effects but they do far more good than harm."

Assessment: 45-year-old man with bipolar disorder with psychotic features who adheres to odd beliefs during periods of stable mood. If there is further evidence of hallucinations during mood-neutral period, then schizoaffective, mixed type is the appropriate diagnosis.

Schizophrenia vs. Schizoaffective Disorder—
Manic Type—CASE STUDY 2.4

Source: Patient and school counselor.

History of present illness: The patient is a 19-year-old male brought in by his school counselor for diagnostic evaluation and consideration of treatment. He describes hearing a voice "when angry." He initially describes this experience since 10 years of age, several months after falling on ice and hitting his head. However, he states that it was not until 15 years of age that he realized they were voices, and later states that the experience is "much worse" since 17–18 years of age. He states he becomes angry when people disrespect him, at which point the voice says things like, "Who does he think he is?" and "Go get him!" When asked, the patient gives a disorganized example of disrespect recalling when a "random person" in the hall said, "Get your brother's jacket off" to a friend. The patient says the random person "knew" she was talking to him, and furthermore that she meant she thought his jacket was too small and must be his brother's. He approached the woman and confronted her, to which she reacted by indicating that she didn't know what he was referring to. He works out at a gym 6 days per week after school and claims to be a formidable boxer, which school officials say is not true. He also plans to invest his tax return in a mutual fund to make money for financial security. He has a history of spending a $150 paycheck all at once. Sleep and appetite are normal.

Medications: None presently; he took olanzapine while in hospital.

Past medical history: No illnesses, fell and hit head once without loss of consciousness, no seizures or neurological disorders.

Psychiatric history: Hospitalized 1-month prior for "3 days," reportedly left against medical advice, no follow-up or meds on discharge.

Social history: High school senior, getting Bs/Cs in regular classes. He was held back in 3rd grade and 5th grade. No drug or alcohol use or history, lives with mother "nanny," stepfather, and two sisters; parents are divorced, and his father has nine other children. He claims to be sexually active with "28 girls"—"one at a time," none presently.

Family history: No history of mental illness.

Mental status exam:

Behavior: Pleasant, cooperative.
Speech: Pressured.
Mood: Good.
Affect: Bright.
Thought process: Circumstantial.
Thought content: Grandiose with referential thinking; no thought insertion or withdrawal; no suicidal, homicidal, or persecutory ideation.
Perception: Auditory hallucinations "when angry" of man's voice commenting and talking to him.
Insight: Fair.
Judgment: Good.

Assessment: 19-year-old male with hallucinations, referential delusions, and thought disorder in the current context of hypomania. Symptoms present by his account since approximately 15 years of age, with exacerbation in past 1–2 years. Symptoms are consistent with a diagnosis of schizophrenia versus schizoaffective disorder. The presence of primarily grandiose delusions would suggest a component of mania. However, on balance suggest schizophrenia.

Recommendation: Resume treatment with an antipsychotic such as olanzapine and follow with psychiatric care.

Schizophrenia vs. Depressive Disorder—CASE STUDY 2.5

Source: The patient is an articulate 42-year-old black woman who is in the care of a resident psychiatrist for "major depression with mild schizophrenia." (Note, although the referring attending psychiatrist used this terminology, no such diagnosis exists.)

History of present illness: The patient describes an episode of depressed mood with poor motivation since she was laid off from her job during a company reorganization at the age of 39. She has been hospitalized twice, and takes Zoloft 50 mg and olanzapine 2.5 mg. She denies any hallucinations or delusions, ever; she has no periods of poor sleep or any other symptom consistent with mania or schizophrenia.

Medication history: Fluoxetine 50 mg/day, reduced from 100 mg previously and Zyprexa 2.5 mg, reduced from 10 mg. She also takes Advir and albuterol but is unable to provide doses.

Past medical history: Asthma and hysterectomy for anemia secondary to endometriosis and fibroids.

Family history: She has two sisters with no significant history of medical or psychiatric illness.

Social history: She lives with father, has no drug use, and drinks one glass of wine every few months.

Mental status exam:

Appearance and behavior: Well dressed, pleasant, articulate, and interpersonally appropriate.
Speech: Normal rate and volume.
Mood: "Better, now that the hysterectomy is behind me."
Affect: Blunted, but appropriate.
Thought process: Logical and linear.
Thought content: No suicidal or homicidal thought, no aggression or delusions.
Perception: No abnormalities now or ever.

Cognition: Difficulty on "serial sevens" (patients are asked to count down from 100 by sevens) and spelling the word "world" backwards (both tasks are done in order to assess concentration). However she will not attempt the latter saying, "I can't do that one."

Insight and judgment: Good.

Assessment: This presentation is most consistent with major depressive disorder versus normal demoralization due to chronic illness and unemployment, status postsurgery with iron deficiency anemia after long course of endometriosis and profuse vaginal bleeding. Mild cognitive impairment appears to me secondary to poor effort. There is no evidence of schizophrenia.

Recommendations: Recommend discontinuation of olanzapine immediately.

Schizophrenia vs. Depressive Disorder—Case Study 2.6

Source: The patient is a 17-year-old white female referred for evaluation following a report of auditory and visual hallucinations.

History of present illness: She relays a 5-year history of seasonal depressed mood without neurovegetative signs (lethargy, somnolence, poor appetite, and poor energy). She states that for several months, in the context of working late at night to finish school papers for graduation, she experienced hearing her name called with no one home. She also relays a one-time experience of hearing the word "tattletale." The patient also states she saw a person standing on the breakers at a pier in Atlantic City and thought it was a visual hallucination. However, she had no corroboration that the person was not there. She denies any delusional content. She received an MRI, EEG, and blood tests, which were all normal except for nonspecific slow spikes on her left temporal EEG without specification of clinical significance.

Past medical history: None.

Medications: None.

Past psychiatric history: She saw a social worker 2 years ago for depressed mood and saw a psychologist in 3rd grade for "waking up her mother at night frequently." She then saw a psychologist again 2 months ago to "resolve depression before going to school." She was then referred to a psychiatrist based on her report of auditory hallucinations, whom she saw twice before this consultation.

Social history: She does not use drugs, is the salutatorian at her high school, is not sexually active, and has many friends. She has been accepted to matriculate at a 4-year college upon graduation from high school.

Family history: She reports multiple uncles, aunts, and cousins that have been treated for depression. She also notes a family history of thyroid disease.

Mental status exam:

Behavior: Pleasant, cooperative.
Speech: Normal.
Mood: "Good."
Affect: Full and appropriate.
Thought process: Logical.
Thought content: Lacks suicidal, homicidal, or delusional content.
Perception: Remarkable for a history of "hearing my name called late at night," and a one time occurrence of hearing a single word, "tattletale." Also note one time when she "saw a person on the breakers" at a beach as noted above, which may have been real.
Insight: Good.
Judgment: Appropriate.
Cognition: Unimpaired during exam and based on performance at school.

Assessment: The patient is a 17-year-old white female with seasonal depressed mood of mild to moderate severity lacking neurovegetative symptoms. Her history is not consistent with a diagnosis of major depressive episodes based on severity or duration. There is no evidence for a psychotic disorder such as schizophrenia or bipolar disorder presently. Rather, she has had isolated, simple illusions or monosyllabic hallucinations in the context of fatigue and stress. These experiences are within the realm of the normal human experience.

Recommendation: No intervention was required, she was advised to follow up with a psychiatrist if her seasonal depression returned or became more severe.

Addendum: Distinguishing characteristics: Characteristic delusions and hallucinations in affective disorders differ from those in schizophrenia. Depressive delusions are generally nonbizarre, self-deprecating, and mood congruent. For example, a depressed patient will typically believe that they have done something bad or are disliked rather than having the types of bizarre and elaborate delusions found in schizophrenia. Alternatively, manic delusions are typically grandiose in nature. For example, manic patients often believe they are especially gifted or important.

Why Does Diagnosis Matter— Implications for Treatment

It is important to distinguish situational demoralization that occurs in the context of negative symptoms of schizophrenia (flat affect and loss of emotion) from an independent affective illness such as major depression. Loss of morale can often occur among people with schizophrenia because they lack friends, meaningful work, joy in life, or prospects of a productive future. Additionally, patients with schizophrenia will often describe their mood as depressed, meaning that they are not happy. Despite these similarities, one should not prescribe antidepressant medication for the demoralization and negative symptoms of schizophrenia. Specifically, although there is clear evidence for the efficacy of antidepressant medications for mood and neurovegetative symptoms in major depressive illness, there is little or no evidence that antidepressants are effective for primary negative symptoms in schizophrenia (Kohler & Martin, 2006;

Lee, Kim, Lee, & Suh, 1998). Furthermore, antidepressants generally constrict patients' range for both positive and negative emotions, meaning they neither feel the full extent of highs or lows. However, schizophrenia patients already have blunted affect, suggesting that further restriction may be counterproductive. Similarly, antipsychotic medications will likely reduce the psychotic component of an affective illness but have little or no efficacy for the mood in major depression. There are also important distinctions regarding the role of psychotherapy. Unlike in schizophrenia, psychotherapy may play a major role in treating underlying illness in depression. However, the mission of psychotherapy in schizophrenia is to help the patient deal with the illness, not treat it. Specifically, psychotherapy has no impact on hallucinations, delusions, disorganization, or primary negative symptoms. However, talk therapy may help the patient learn how to manage symptoms and interact more productively within society. This is analogous to the use of psychotherapy in cancer patients, where the primary tumor requires medication or radiation, and psychotherapy can help deal with the impact of cancer on the patient's daily life and future.

Negative Symptoms vs. Neurovegetative Signs of Depression—CASE STUDY 2.7

Source: Patient interview.

Chief complaint: "I am not able to do the things I am supposed to or want to."

History of present illness: The patient is a 33-year-old Hispanic male who is primarily upset over not attaining his life goals and failing to achieve his own and family's expectations. He is living in his family's apartment in his native country, where he sees a therapist weekly. He is unemployed and has completed 1 year of college in Guatemala as well as "90 credit hours" at a college in Texas where he received *D*s and *C*s. He describes college performance as "poor" secondary to poor effort and planning, often procrastinating, choosing to spend time socially, or visiting the city rather than working. He has participated in several "groups" over the past 4 years, which he found especially helpful in their ability to lend support from people with similar problems. Presently he cannot have group therapy in Guatemala and hopes to return to the United States to obtain it. However, his mother will no longer pay to send him to the United States to continue failing in school and has "insisted I get a job and show her that I can be responsible." The patient feels pressured by his mother and complains she is too controlling, despite understanding why she has become frustrated with him. He hopes to return to college, obtain an undergraduate degree in business, and then a master's degree in psychology to pursue a career in business psychology and organizational psychology.

Review of systems: He complains of increased sleep during the day with difficulty sleeping at night, appetite is good with 35 lb weight gain over "a long time," as well as tearfulness. No anhedonia or alogia.

Past medical history: Hypertrigliceridemia.

Psychiatric history:

1. Diagnosis of dysthymic disorder with possible episode of major depression—treated at approximately 16 years of age with tonfranil and recently with Prozac 20 mg po qd × 4 months without efficacy according to patient and records.
2. Diagnosis of schizophrenia—with "only negative symptoms" by records—treated previously with risperidone 6 mg per day and olanzapine, both "without improvement."
3. Prior diagnosis of avoidant personality disorder.
4. Treated as outpatient for 1 year with individual psychotherapy and cognitive therapy in Guatemala, which he enjoys.
5. IQ test in 1997—115 according to patient's report.

Family history: Paternal alcohol abuse; maternal grandfather—bipolar disorder.

Social history: Denies current substance use, remote history of social alcohol, lives in an apartment that is owned by his mother, is the oldest of three brothers, and has made repeated attempts at college without success.

Mental status exam:

Behavior: Pleasant, cooperative 33-year-old male appropriately dressed.
Speech: Normal.
Mood: "Depressed, close to tears when thinking about sad things."
Affect: Full and appropriately responsive.
Thought process: Logical and well organized.
Thought content: Without suicidal or aggressive thoughts or intent.
Perception: Denies abnormalities.
Insight: Good: "I understand why my mother has lost hope in me, and I understand that I have to earn her confidence back before returning to school."
Judgment: Fair: "I still want to return to the United States for 1 month of group therapy, even though I know my mother won't pay for it and I have no other means to do so."

MRI: Normal brain image.

Labs: Complete blood count, chemistry profile, thyroid functions all within normal range, triglycerides—688 (25–50), lipid profile otherwise within normal range.

Assessment: Patient is a 33-year-old male with approximately 17-year history of psychiatric contact since the divorce of his parents. During that period he has experienced difficulty attaining his educational, social, and vocational goals due to a variety of factors including poor motivation and organizational skills and likely periods of dysthymic disorder and episodes of major depression interspersed with euthymia. Despite having received a previous diagnosis of schizophrenia based on "predominantly negative symptoms," there is no evidence to support this diagnosis. Specifically, the patient lacks thought disorder, alogia, or any positive symptoms either now or previously. Additionally, there is no evidence for bipolar disorder either presently or by history.

Recommendations:

1. Pharmacotherapy for dysthymic disorder with Wellbutrin, which is less likely to be associated with risk of weight gain; initial dose 100 mg po qd then increase to 100 mg bid with a final dose of 150 mg po bid over approximately 2 weeks.
2. Continue individual psychotherapy with involvement of his mother and other family members to discuss relational issues of control and dependence that are pertinent to patient's situation.
3. Continue online chat group with members of former group therapy to obtain social supports of "people like me" in absence of ability to return to group therapy in the United States.

■ Schizophrenia vs. Anxiety Disorders—CASE STUDY 2.8

Source: Patient, parents, and records.

History of present illness: The patient is a 24-year-old male who was discharged from a community hospital the day prior to evaluation. He was voluntarily hospitalized 1 week ago, secondary to thoughts of self-harm with subjective depression and hopelessness. He describes feeling a sense of increasing sadness and isolation since a neuropsychological evaluation several months ago. That test concluded that the patient has "schizophrenia." The patient and his parents state they were devastated by the diagnosis. Other results indicate above-average performance with a full-scale IQ of 113 and verbal IQ of 118.

The patient states he had a normal childhood, following birth by emergent Cesarean section. He did well in school, receiving "*As* and *Bs*" in high school. He states he had friends, including a "best friend" whom he can name (requiring a name is often used to distinguish true friends versus acquaintances or strangers). However, he states he was not as close with people as he believes others are. After high school, he attended college for 1 year. During that year, he states he did not work hard enough and decided not to return as he was, "wasting my parent's money." Additionally, he had one episode of unusual behavior in which he struck his roommate in the face for "smoking in the room and refusing to stop." He then attended vocational school for 3 months during the following year, during which he had a second incident of aggression. At that time he struck his roommate in a dispute over the TV remote. Neither incident resulted in legal action or medical care. The patient left school and joined the Navy, where he served without difficulties as a petty officer on a submarine for 4 years. During that period, he states he enjoyed the structure and was able meet the requirements of the job. However, toward the end of his tour of duty, he states he became upset over a relationship with a girl who stated that he "did not talk enough." He mentioned his sadness to his parents, but preferred not to seek treatment in the Navy out of concern that it would tarnish his record. He received an honorable discharge and proceeded to work full time after leaving the military. He currently works 40 hours per week.

He received counseling for sadness including treatment with Zoloft for 1 month, which was changed to Paxil by his family physician. While living apart from his parents, he became increasingly depressed and requested that they pick him up since he was scared he would harm himself. Following the neuropsychological testing (noted above), he has been in treatment with a psychiatrist who prescribed risperidone 4 mg/day, lithium 300 mg/day, and Effexor 150 mg/day. Approximately 1 week prior to hospitalization, Effexor was changed to Paxil. He states medication had no effect. His parents concur, with the exception that, "He may have been a little calmer."

The patient has gained 30 lb over the past 6 months, which he attributes to medication. Upon discharge from hospital, his medications have been changed to Prozac in place of Paxil, and olanzapine 10 mg per day in place of risperidone. The patient and his parents state that the change to olanzapine was "due to the weight gain." (Authors' note: This is paradoxical since olanzapine is generally associated with much greater weight gain than risperidone).

He describes periods of rapid onset pounding heart, sweating, and "panic," which never happen at home, but often happen in public places (3–4 times per week). He states he also has had extreme sweating all his life, even when calm, and has arranged for a sympathectomy at a university hospital 1 week after this evaluation.

Mental status exam:

Behavior: Pleasant with intermittent eye contact.

Speech: Normal.

Mood: "Anxious" and "upset."

Affect: Restricted but appropriate with periods of expressed emotion (smiling).

Thought process: Logical without evidence of thought disorder.

Thought content: He denies current thoughts of self-harm or harm to others. He states that at times he has had a vague sense that people wanted to harm him, but no concrete delusions.

Perception: No abnormalities. However, he describes "hearing his family, like a memory, but I can tell who it is." He states this experience is different than actually hearing someone talk, and he has never looked for a source, as it is "clearly inside my head."

Insight: Good: "I want to be with people, but I have a hard time interacting with them."

Judgment: Good: "I thought I would hurt myself, so I called my parents and asked for help."

Cognition: Concentration is fair, becoming distracted occasionally, "when the other person talks a lot."

Assessment: The patient is a 24-year-old man with medical history consistent with social phobia, anxiety, and periods of depression.

There is no evidence of frank psychosis or thought disorder. His history is not consistent with a diagnosis of schizophrenia at this time.

Recommendation: Given the paucity of evidence for a psychotic process, it is recommended that antipsychotic medication be terminated under the supervision of a treating psychiatrist. It is further recommended that treatment concentrate on his anxiety/ depressive symptoms with consideration of a diagnosis of social phobia versus generalized anxiety with agoraphobia.

■ Schizophrenia vs. Obsessive-Compulsive Disorder—
CASE STUDY 2.9

Source: Patient and records.

History of present illness: Patient is a 21-year-old white male who initially reports 1.5 years of symptoms that began in college. He is currently between junior and senior year. The patient has not taken any time off from school. He states that while a sophomore, he began having trouble thinking and headaches, thus concluding that he was loosing brain cells. During this time he was aggressive toward many people, frequently "giving them the finger" in a compulsive manner. Although he did not report this to me, he told others that he had to give everyone the finger to stop from loosing brain cells. The patient also complained of blurry vision at that time for which an eye doctor could find no cause and which resolved on antipsychotic medication. He states he ran the bases naked at school and masturbated in public at the library, neither of which he thinks were odd. His mother reports he was disorganized, at times with unintelligible speech. She also reports that he threatened to stab her in the genitals (using an inappropriately vernacular term for one's mother). The patient did not mention that, but he did report intermittent, fleeting thoughts of wanting to kill his father. He is very clear he has no intention to ever act on these thoughts and realizes they are not acceptable.

There is no history of sleep disturbances, gambling, excessive spending, or promiscuity. He did report "speaking fast and having fast thoughts." No evidence of grandiosity. For example, he stated he wants to be a professional tennis player, but was quick to add, "That is what I want, although I know it's not realistic, so I'll try to get a government job since my dad says they get really good benefits."

Despite his initial report that it all began in college, he reports depression and suicidality lasting "for 3 years" in high school after the death of an acquaintance. He also reports that he used to rub his leg up against girls inappropriately, although this has only resulted in one girl telling him to "go away" (using the appropriate vernacular for his age). No history of incarceration. He states that he is often concerned that someone will beat him up, which he attributes to having been beaten up in high school after making fun of a kid with Tourette's syndrome. He states the kid did not react appropriately to his teasing. He considers reacting appropriately "not trying to kill me."

Social history: He states he has two friends at home and two to three at school, whom he sees at least several times per week. He is currently working full time (last 6 days), having lost a previous job. He also reports working out daily with a friend, except when working full time. He has one younger sister. He does not use any drugs or alcohol.

Family history: Significant for affective illness on both sides—maternal grandmother committed suicide.

Medications: Trileptal, aripiprazole, hydroxyzine, and Anafranil.

Mental status exam:

Behavior: Pleasant, cooperative.
Speech: Normal.
Mood: Good.
Affect: Full.
Thought process: Logical and linear.
Thought content: Denies current suicidal ideation (SI), but states that at times he thinks of dying because he is bored. Denies

current homicidal ideation (HI), but has intermittent thoughts to kill father over past perceived slight, "He pulled on my ID string when I wouldn't help him install a stereo in my dorm room." Insight and judgment are impaired; he minimizes the implications of his past behaviors.

Perception: Denies current or past abnormalities (although his report of blurry vision may be a perceptual distortion).

Insight: Poor at times, such as other child's reaction to teasing.

Judgment: Poor—masturbating in the library.

Assessment: 21-year-old male with obsessive behaviors (the finger) driven by fear of consequences (loosing brain cells) with history of depressed mood and aggressive, inappropriate behaviors consistent with poor executive function and frontal lobe signs (masturbating in public, running naked in public, rubbing up against girls in college and high school). He has features consistent with:

- Obsessive-compulsive disorder (OCD)—behaviors driven by anxiety and consequences.
- Bipolar disorder, type 1/mixed—fast thoughts and fast speech as well as periods of depression preceding psychosis.
- Schizophrenia—Supported by delusion of loosing brain cells, disorganized thoughts and behaviors. However, he lacks negative symptoms or hallucinations, lacking full criteria. Given his young age, it is also possible that he is experiencing early, prodromal signs of schizophrenia with OCD features.

Recommendation: Given the diagnostic uncertainty, it would be better to target one disease as the primary cause of his difficulties. One could then evaluate efficacy based on treatment of the primary etiology before adding multiple medications. For example, he could be treated for OCD using Anafranil while discontinuing Trileptal, aripiprazole, and hydroxyzine. If he develops further signs of delusional thought or true hallucinations, an antipsychotic agent could be added. If, however, frontal release behaviors persist, agents such as valproate may be helpful for impulse control.

Schizophrenia vs. Developmental Disorder—CASE STUDY 2.10

Sources: Patient, both parents, records.

History of present illness: The patient is an 18-year-old male currently in the 12th grade. He and his family describe approximately 1-year history of obsession with a girl he knows resulting in a court order and arrest related to persistent efforts to contact her. They describe him as a child that has always been a loner, with an unusual propensity to do whatever he was asked, despite a complete lack of internal motivation. As an example, they site he has always gotten straight *A*'s in school but has no desire to go to college. In fact, he threw out solicitations to Ivy League colleges and asked that his parents choose a school for him if he must go to one. He will therefore go to a local college to enable him to remain at home, in accordance with medical advice they have received. They add that he has had a few friends, all of whom have been related to him. However, "Once his cousin walks out of the room, (the patient) will not give him another minute's thought for a year." The patient describes that he craves human closeness but cannot achieve it. He states he has been profoundly depressed for a year, with multiple hospitalizations and two suicide notes in the last 2 weeks. They add he can sleep up to 16 hours per day, but that has improved since he began both Effexor (225 mg) and Geodon (60 mg bid). His mother states there had been no such improvement on multiple trials of SSRIs previously, also noting that the antipsychotic medication Navane did nothing either.

He denies any history of auditory hallucinations. Delusions are not clear. He states he does not feel pain, but qualifies this to mean he has become desensitized. He states he can punch a nail through his hand without feeling it. His parents say this has come up in the past, but that no mark remains when he shows them. Other possible delusions are limited to instances of extremely poor insight and judgment including, "I think it would help to talk to (the woman's name omitted) to bring closure," despite clear admonition from his treating psychiatrist that this would be a very bad idea.

Medication history: He is compliant with medication, currently on Effexor 225 mg/day and Geodon 60 mg bid. He was previously treated with Navane for 2 weeks, and has had multiple trials of antidepressants. The patient reported that all of these medications made him feel worse. His mother adds that the previous medications did not lead to any improvement. He is also taking Propecia for hair loss.

Past medical history: Premature birth and motor delay by record and premature hair loss. Previous psychiatric diagnoses include major depressive disorder and psychosis not otherwise specified (NOS).

Family history: He has two affected cousins by report, with one who completed suicide.

Social history: No history of drug use, few social contacts, and no romantic relationships. He has been arrested and has a restraining order related to menacing (name omitted). He has been charged with pornography and admits to buying adult material (pornographic magazine) at a legal store. Parents concur that there does not appear to be a real legal violation in regard to that specific charge. His family notes that his complete lack of interest in activities that typically get teenage boys in trouble was seen as a blessing until recently. He does watch movies over and over, and plays Dungeons and Dragons with friends. His father notes that he "comes back to life" when his friends come over to play, then "collapses for 16 hours like it exhausted him." He states there is nothing that makes him happy and nothing he wants to do. As an example, he is willing to go to college but sees no difference between that path and watching TV instead. Also, they say he was appropriately social in some contexts; for example, he would play appropriately on little league team but never wanted teammates to come over to play.

Mental status exam:

Appearance and behavior: Poor eye contact, no aggression, at end of interview he stood and faced the wall until his father pointed out that it was inappropriate. He smiled and said that it was as much of the interview as he could take (after about 1–1.5 hours). Possible akathisia (restlessness; see page 161) noted; however, he smiled at the notion that it annoyed his parents and he could do it since it might be related to his medications. Generally quite pleasant and cooperative during exam, although very passive, preferring to have his parents relay the story.

Speech: Normal, with decreased amount.

Mood: Depressed, crying daily, "empty."

Affect: Blunted to flat, with two smiles over the course of lengthy interview.

Thought process: Linear, logical, although disconnected emotionally— for example, acknowledges but does not understand that his suicide would hurt his parents. Although there is no evidence of thought disorder, a letter in his chart has a few neologisms intercalated in a very articulate description of an internal psychological "battle" between the "boy and the beast" in his mind.

Thought content: No delusions beyond the self-described desensitization "I don't feel pain." Clear obsession with (name omitted), still adhering to hope that he will speak to her and reinforcing that if she goes to college without speaking to him, there will be no reason to live. He continues to endorse suicidal ideation, with no plan. He has an appointment with his psychiatrist shortly, and his parents say they are aware of his intentions, as well as the increased risk of completion in his "mildly improved" state.

Perception: No auditory hallucinations or other perceptual abnormalities, "like actually hearing a voice." He does initially state he heard voices, but clarifies to mean ruminations of his own thoughts and voice in his head during a dizzy episode.

Cognition: Records indicate an IQ in the "140 range." He continues to achieve all *A*'s presently in high school.

Insight and judgment: Extremely poor. He demonstrates no sign of acknowledging that suicide is not an appropriate solution to his despair over (name omitted). He states that she is the first person in life he felt connected to and that he fears he can not recreate that, given his relative social discomfort and awkwardness. As such, he has concluded that life is not worth living without her. He clearly states he will not act on these thoughts until (name omitted) has left for college. His family is planning to be with him at that time, having arranged leave of work, and considering a trip to remove him from the environment.

Assessment: Most consistent with major depressive episode. Records state that he received a previous diagnosis of psychosis not otherwise specified (NOS), considering schizophrenia vs. depression with psychotic features. He clearly has depressed mood, anhedonia, poor motivation, and poor insight. All but the subjective sense of sadness could be equally attributed to negative symptoms as they can to depression. There is little to currently support psychosis, with the caveat that he is on Geodon. However, there is also little to support previous psychosis, aside from an irrational obsessive preoccupation with a "first love" and very poor judgment in response to her rejection. One cannot rule out a prodrome for psychotic processes, but affective illness with severe premorbid social difficulties cannot be dismissed either. His craving of human contact, despite his inability to attain it, argues more for Asperger's spectrum developmental disorder than schizoid personality. He was not evaluated for developmental disorders as a child because there were no problems that raised that level of concern at the time.

■ Prodromal Schizophrenia vs. Pervasive Developmental Disorder—CASE STUDY 2.11

Source: Patient and parents.

History of present illness: Patient is a 19-year-old male seen in the presence of his mother for diagnostic evaluation. Prior records were reviewed. Patient and his mother describe a history that is entirely consistent with the comprehensive notes and summary of prior psychiatrist. Pertinent highlights follow.

Patient was expelled from college for odd behavior including making inappropriate jokes and a bizarre interaction with his professor. He describes wanting to be a great comedian and continues presently to endorse this desire. He also focuses on smiling as a way to overcome depression. He is socially isolated, both because of a profound difficulty connecting with people and because his approach to socializing makes him an outcast owing to the inappropriate nature of his actions. He does not seem to be able to, or conversely want to, cease all unsuccessful social strategies such as telling jokes. He has been hospitalized twice. He has received diagnoses of schizoaffective disorder as well as medication for both psychosis and depression. Although there is evidence of a mood disorder, including his subjective report of not being happy for long periods of time, they are not consistent or complete evidence to support frank bipolar disorder or schizophrenia. Specifically, he has:

1. Experienced occupational decline due to odd behavior and inappropriate social strategies. While odd, his behavior is not disorganized.
2. Displayed odd (smiling) and/or restricted affect.
3. Described periods of suicidal ideation.
4. Displayed odd, if not grandiose, thoughts of becoming the greatest comedian.
5. Inconsistent cognitive capabilities, characterized by average intelligence with rapid speed and poor memory for some types of stimuli.
6. Unusual motor tics and verbalizations.

He has not:

1. Had frank delusions or hallucinations
2. Had periods of clear mania (boundless energy, wild spending sprees, dangerous and/or reckless behavior) or classical major depression (persistent anhedonia, crying, worthlessness, and

neurovegetative signs such as weight loss, insomnia, or leaden paralysis).

Family history: Remarkable for both schizophrenia (grandmother and brother) and autism. His mother also reports affective/anxiety spectrum disorders including an eating disorder.

Medical history: Remarkable for pericarditis with an effusion at age 17.

Psychiatric history: As noted, he has been treated for affective and psychotic disorders but lacks a full spectrum of symptoms to support either.

Developmental history: Remarkable for extra help, but not special education, in grade school as well as periods of holding his breath "until passing out" as a child.

Social history: He describes having friends as a child. His parents divorced when he was young. Patient currently lives with his father. His mother describes his father as being very supportive of him recently since his difficulties escalated in college.

Mental status exam:

Behavior: Patient was pleasant and cooperative with no signs of aggression or disorganized behavior.

Appearance: Normally dressed and in no apparent distress, age and situationally appropriate.

Speech: No signs of pressured or labored speech; normal prosody and volume.

Affect: Slightly odd, smiling at times to demonstrate his strategy for maintaining a positive mood.

Mood: Sad at times, but also able to feel happy on occasion.

Thought process: Linear and logical without evidence of gross disorganization.

Thought content: No suicidal or aggressive/homicidal thoughts. No frank delusions of persecution or reference. He does continue to adhere to a grandiose aspiration to become a great stand-up comedian. He does not think he is a great comedian yet, but lacks the insight or judgment to realize how ineffective this plan is, and how unlikely it is for him to achieve this goal.

Perception: No hallucinations of any kind.

Insight: Very poor; he lacks the basic understanding of how his own behavior propagated and exacerbates his difficulty.

Judgment: Equally poor; he continues to practice his "routine" and smiling oddly as a social strategy.

Cognition: Formal testing not performed; however, comprehensive testing records indicate average intelligence and capabilities.

Assessment: Patient is a 19-year-old male with an unusual constellation of strange, and ultimately self-destructive, behaviors that have clearly risen to the level of medical attention due to consequences including being removed from class by police and expelled from college. Additionally, his pattern of interpersonal strategies and behavior further alienate him from friends and society at large. However, he lacks a consistent or coherent picture for any one psychiatric disorder, prompting appropriate concern that he may be in the prodromal stages of developing either schizophrenia or bipolar disorder. He has received several psychiatric medications including risperidone, aripiprazole, Prozac, and Effexor. These appear more driven by disability and the desire to "do something" than any clear evidence based on specific symptoms. It is not clear to me that medication is in fact indicated. However, given his family history, decline in function, and preponderance of odd behaviors, continued observation is appropriate. Suggestion of symptoms should be carefully avoided, as he could start endorsing symptoms if he perceives that he is "supposed" to have them. Asperger's syndrome, characterized by relatively preserved cognition with profound difficulty in social interactions, is among the better fitting diagnoses. Given his strong desire for social interactions, autism is less consistent among the developmental disorders.

Recommendations: I do not see a role for medications presently, and use of potential stimulants such as aripiprazole may actually exacerbate, rather than ameliorate, the situation. If he does take antidepressants, I suggest relatively calming, rather than activating types (avoid bupropion) and being vigilant for drug-induced mania. Similarly, if antipsychotics are prescribed for behavioral control, I suggest avoiding medications that can become activating at high doses, like aripiprazole. Quetiapine is generally more effective as a calming, prosleep agent and has a relatively benign side effect profile. As in the case for this patient, where the evidence for the need for any medication is weak, a mild, safe medication like quetiapine may be most appropriate. If, however, antipsychotic efficacy becomes needed, I suggest the use of risperidone, olanzapine, or any number of older, quite effective medications such as haloperidol, trifluoperazine, or perphenazine. None of these are indicated presently. Mostly, the patient appears to need social skills training. He needs to embrace change and give up his attempts to engage society through comedy. These behavioral changes should, in my opinion, be the focus of therapy so he can integrate into an age-appropriate group and complete college.

Substance-Induced Disorders to Distinguish from Schizophrenia

Substance-Induced Psychosis—Medication or Illicit Drug—CASE STUDY 2.12

Source: Parents and patient.

History of present illness: The patient is a 16-year-old male. He and his parents noted a change in behavior during 8th grade. He experienced periods of sadness at that time, but not consistently. Despite this feeling, he continued all normal activities in and around school. Of note, they went on a family trip abroad the previous summer during which he was "bored," and returned early. They also note one incident of extreme irritability at that time coupled with increased sleep, and periods of inactivity initially upon his return to the United States. He later returned to a more normal pattern of activity.

He then began high school, at which time they note he appeared more depressed. He had a great deal of difficulty dealing with the increased pressure and need to navigate the new building more quickly. He had an individualized educational plan (IEP) since 1st grade based on his slower speed of performing some activities. However, he made new friends, tried out for two school sport teams, and was playing guitar. He was cut from one of the sports teams, which his parents describe as devastating for him. He also began trying marijuana, which he estimates as less than 10 times, opium about three times, and drinking alcohol with these new friends. During that winter, he became intoxicated while spending time with a group of older students. The patient was picked up by police and had his driving license eligibility delayed, as a result.

During that period he also had more colds and fell behind in school. His parents note that he began Accutane for acne around that same period, which was his second round of treatment. That finished after 7 months of treatment. He did not ever experience hallucinations, but did express concern that people were angry at him and were talking about him at school, which is the closest he comes to experiencing a delusion.

There was an acute episode that brought him to clinical attention. He "escaped" from class to go to the bathroom and told a stranger there that he was concerned he had become addicted to an opiate and that he did not feel well. His parents note that the incident was preceded by 3–4 days without any sleep and some weight loss. He had also used an opiate narcotic one time a few days earlier. His family has been told that he might have been in withdrawal, despite the very limited use and long latency to the acute incident. He was taken to their local community hospital where he had a clean drug screen and was diagnosed with anxiety. He then saw a community psychiatrist one time, who prescribed trazadone 50 mg, presumably for sleep. After the incident at school, he left public high school and now attends private school.

Developmental history: As noted above, the patient has an IEP in place since 1st grade to accommodate longer time required for some tasks.

Medical history: Acne, treated with Accutane on two occasions for approximately 6–8 months.

Social history: As noted above, he has several friends, has tried marijuana, opium, and alcohol, but has no history of intravenous drug use. He lives with his parents and has one older and one younger sibling. His older sibling had a substance use problem in high school as well, but is applying for college presently.

Medication: None presently. Previously, he was treated with Accutane for acne, Ativan for anxiety, trazadone for sleep, and risperidone 0.5 to 1 mg for psychotic disorder NOS briefly for 2 months.

Family history: His grandmother attempted suicide in her 40s and developed Alzheimer's disease with psychosis later in life. A grandfather may have been depressed, but never had formal diagnosis; one of his aunts was thought to have had postpartum depression.

Mental status exam:

Appearance: Normal grooming and hygiene in age-appropriate clothing.
Behavior: Initially appeared bewildered or mildly disoriented, which became less pronounced throughout the interview.
Speech: Normal volume and prosody, with minimal amount.
Mood: "OK."
Affect: Restricted, but engaged, within normal range for a teenager in this situation.
Thought process: Linear and logical.
Thought content: No suicidal or aggressive thoughts, no delusions.
Perception: No hallucinations.

Insight: Good, appeared open to the idea that he needed to stop all complicating behaviors such as drug and alcohol use.

Judgment: Reasonable; he was willing to come for evaluation and has shared information with his parents.

Impulse control: No difficulties.

Cognition: Within normal range based on general interview; no formal testing done at this time. Records indicate baseline IQ of approximately 115. School performance has been slightly lower than one might anticipate with that score. He has been diagnosed with and received accommodation for a learning disability.

Assessment: Although the patient has been diagnosed with psychotic disorder NOS and "first break psychosis" in past, I am hesitant to conclude he has a bona fide, biological disorder. Rather, I think his substance use complicates interpretation, especially in the context of his adjustment to high school.

One possibility is that his emotional/affective symptoms and minimal psychotic experience may have resulted from exposure to Accutane, as both are described among its adverse reactions, albeit not common ones.

Presently he appears neither depressed nor psychotic.

Recommendations: Stop using all drugs and alcohol. Never resume the drug use, be careful with the alcohol after age 21, if then. Failure to heed this warning will continue to complicate interpretation, lead to continued exposure to medications such as risperidone to counter the effects of substance abuse, and marginalize him from the healthcare system, which generally is less sympathetic and engaged with substance abusers than people with bona fide illness.

Accutane has already been stopped. I would not recommend resuming it in the future based on a possible link to his symptoms.

Continue to work with his outpatient psychiatrist and his school district to help patient meet the demands of high school without as many unnecessary additional stressors as possible. He should first master his required activities before engaging in too many extracurricular ones.

Ultimately it will be best for him to reintegrate into the mainstream high school where he can regain a sense of normalcy and return to his original life trajectory.

Personality Disorders to Distinguish from Schizophrenia

Prior to describing an example of how personality can confound diagnosis, it is important to describe personality disorders in detail. Personality disorders are characterized by a pattern of maladaptive behaviors, perceptions, and interactions that are stable and cross personal, social, and occupational domains. These patterns of behavior begin in early adulthood and may affect cognition, impulse control, and interpersonal interactions. Although some features of personality disorder can overlap with features of major illnesses, they are milder in both extent and impact. That is, they are mild versions of psychiatric symptoms that generally do not rise to cause the level of impairments seen with schizophrenia or other axis I (i.e., major) disorders. Thus some patients with personality disorders can have attenuated features of schizophrenia. Personality disorders are divided into three main clusters that align along the subdivisions of serious psychiatric disorders as illustrated below.

Clusters

Cluster A

Cluster A is the schizophrenia spectrum. As noted above, cluster A includes three specific subtypes. **Paranoid personality disorder (PD)** patients are suspicious and distrustful while **schizotypal PD** patients tend to be odd or eccentric. Thus, these two subtypes embody mild versions of positive symptoms. Some examples are a strong belief in astrology and magic numbers or extreme suspiciousness in a person that is able to work and have relationships. **Schizoid PD** patients are loners and are emotionally detached with autistic behaviors. These people avoid interpersonal contact and gravitate to solitary jobs such as night watchmen. This group of patients are most similar to schizophrenia, with the major distinction that they are able to function and do not have bizarre delusions (outside of those that are culturally acceptable) or hallucinations.

Cluster B

Cluster B is the affective spectrum. This cluster of disorders is also divided into three subgroups. **Antisocial PD** patients are violent and malevolent with behaviors that harm others. Many of these people were diagnosed with conduct disorder as children. While some people with schizophrenia may become violent due to psychotic content (e.g., "he was sending gamma rays at my genitals so *I knocked him down*"), antisocial PD patients engage in violence for personal gain ("I wanted his money so *I knocked him down* and took it"). **Borderline PD** patients have unstable relationships with alternating periods of overvaluing and devaluing other people. The resulting isolation and perception of betrayal can exacerbate depressed mood, continuing a cycle of low self-esteem. Thus, their solitude and sense of persecution tend to result from reactive or manipulative behaviors rather than a lack of social desire. Additionally, borderline patients' sense of persecution is similar in quality to persecutory delusions of schizophrenia, but is used as a psychological defense to explain why no one likes them. **Histrionic PD** patients are overly dramatic and attention seeking. Thus, they may have mild grandiosity, albeit not rising to the level of delusions in psychotic disorders. Similarly, **narcissistic PD** patients are self-centered and have a high degree of entitlement with lack of empathy. Schizophrenia patients often relate neutral events to themselves, such as, "Everyone is watching me and sending the pictures to the government to harm me." Alternatively, narcissistic PD patients believe that the attention is positive: "I think that woman is looking at me because I'm so attractive."

Cluster C

Cluster C is the anxiety spectrum. These patients exhibit mild versions of anxiety disorders. **Avoidant PD** patients avoid social situations due to social anxiety. Alternatively, schizophrenia patients with prominent negative symptoms tend not to crave human interactions. **Dependent PD** patients are clingy and submissive, with a childlike immaturity. Although schizophrenia patients are often highly dependent on others, this results from a true lack of capability. **Obsessive-compulsive PD** patients are preoccupied with rules and detail. Similarly, schizophrenia patients tend to be very rigid and lack mental flexibility, perhaps due to the overwhelming nature of even minor changes. The distinguishing characteristic is that obsessive-compulsive PD patients can use their adherence to rules within the confines of society.

Disentangling Axis I and Axis II Disorders—Case Study 2.13

Source: The patient is a 17-year-old female referred for clinical consultation regarding diagnosis and treatment recommendations.

History of present illness: The patient reports normal developmental milestones until age 10, when she reports onset of visual and auditory hallucinations related to an elementary school teacher. She states she would see and hear him in her home, but never disclosed this to her family, as she states she thought it was normal. However, her parents add that a peer states that the patient has been talking about hearing voices since 4th grade. The patient states there was never any incident with that teacher and that his being the subject of her hallucinations is apparently random and bewildering. She states that other voices later joined, often in the form of conversations, which were less well articulated than the teacher's. She characterizes voices as indistinguishable from real ones and states she could not distinguish visual hallucinations of that teacher from an actual person.

The patient states that her auditory and visual hallucinations were generally of a pleasant and supportive nature from 10–16 years of age, but that the content became derogatory and threatening after an incident in her midteens. She states she was raped by a male friend while at a party. She stated they were friends and that he approached her while they were alone in a room, but she had not consented to sex. He called her after the incident and she reports that he was unaware that she had not considered it consensual and asked if she was upset about what they had done. She had her phone number changed, eventually disclosed the event to her parents and long-standing boyfriend but did not notify police or press charges. She states that everything has taken a turn for the worse since then.

She was eventually admitted to a psychiatric hospital following an episode at a friend's home when she acted oddly, insisting her friend was not real after which she laid down on his lawn. She also reported to the friend and his father that she had been kicked out of her home by her parents, which was not the case. She continued to state she lived in her car for 1 week after being "put out," but acknowledged that no one else agrees that these events (being kicked out of her home or living in a car) ever occurred.

She is uncomfortable around people and states she has always shied away from crowds. She has one close male friend and an older boyfriend (she says 2 years, records indicate 4 years older). She states they have dated for 2.5 years and that they are sexually active. However, she adds that she does not enjoy time with him or anyone else. She stated her mood had been depressed for at least 6 months and feels like killing herself. She adds that she has no intention of actually hurting herself, beyond cutting, which she has done on a few occasions, "to hurt or punish myself," later adding, "I like blood." She notes that cutting has been motivated by nondepressive, nonpsychotic reasons at times.

She describes herself as an *A* student through most of her academic career, but did poorly on the SAT. Also, her grades deteriorated, which she attributed to missing school for hospitalization and hearing voices. The latter contradicts her statement that voices have been there as long as she can remember.

She started risperidone after first seeing a psychiatrist, noting that it made the voices stop. However, she began to lactate, had an elevated prolactin level, and developed motor side effects. She was then changed to Geodon, at which time the voices resumed. Upon reinitiating risperidone, the voices stopped again after about 1 week. She is also receiving Klonopin and Xanax for anxiety and Prozac for depression as well as Cogentin for the motor side effects of risperidone. She states her mood is still depressed, crying daily with no sense of enjoyment. Sleep is normal, with decreased appetite leading to 20 lb weight loss. She is approximately 150 pounds, 5′ 8″ at this time.

Social history: Patient is a high school senior and was accepted to college. She has one close friend and a boyfriend that is in college. She states she has a good relationship with her parents, but less so with her younger sibling. Records indicate she used marijuana approximately once a month in the past. She has not used any in 2 months.

Medical history: No medical diagnoses. Neurological exam, MRI, and EEG all normal, with possible nonspecific, nonsignificant medication effects on EEG.

Family history: She was adopted with no information available regarding her genetic risk factors. She lives with her parents and younger sibling. She has good relationships with both parents and acknowledges that any conflict they have had related to controlling her activities is motivated by their concern for her well-being.

Mental status exam:

Behavior: Pleasant, appropriate, and cooperative with good eye contact throughout the 3-hour interview. She looked about the room at times, adding, "I thought someone was there."

Speech: Contains normal amount and latency of response.

Mood: Depressed.

Affect: Congruent, mildly restricted but appropriate and responsive during the interview.

Thought process: Linear and well organized.

Thought content: Remarkable for passive suicidal ideation with no intent or plan, no homicidal ideation or thoughts of aggression toward others. Delusions include the incident of being "put out" of her home and living in a car, which never occurred. She also reports being concerned that her friend can put thoughts into her head and that it feels like people can read her thoughts, which she recognizes is not possible.

Perception: Remarkable for previous auditory, visual, olfactory, and tactile hallucinations "since 10 years old." She states she can smell burning when others say it is not there and "was holding a puppy that I could see and feel in the hospital."

Insight: Fair, as she was able to discuss the implausibility of some of her reports and tolerated a frank discussion regarding the possibility she is embellishing or even fabricating some of it.

Judgment: Fair, as evidenced by taking medication and stopping other complicating behaviors such as drug use.

Mini mental status exam: She lost two points for month and day, reporting "February 28" on March 8. Given her overall demeanor and performance on the remainder of the exam, it seems improbable that this was a real attempt, reducing reliability of the test.

Assessment: The patient is a 17-year-old adopted white female reporting psychotic symptoms including polymodal hallucinations, possible delusions of living in her car, very mild persecutory ideation, and ambiguity about thought insertion. Hallucinations appear responsive to appropriate treatment with risperidone, arguing that they are real. However, the polymodal nature of her hallucinations, including auditory, olfactory, visual, and tactile experiences is implausible, suggesting an element of embellishment. She also describes depressed mood with tearfulness, arguing for an affective illness rather than negative symptoms. She displayed self-injurious behavior of a nonpsychotic nature including cutting, suggesting borderline personality features. However, at 17 she remains too young for a diagnosis of borderline personality disorder and does have stable relationships with parents and a boyfriend, also arguing against such a diagnosis. Records indicate monthly marijuana use. Her cognitive function is intact.

Differential diagnosis: She previously received a diagnosis of schizoaffective disorder, supported by auditory hallucinations and depressed mood. Although the patient also exhibits borderline behaviors, such as cutting and likely embellishment of symptoms, it remains premature to make an axis II diagnosis based on her age. The potential role of drug use is not clear, as she declined to elaborate. She has normal EEG, MRI, and comprehensive laboratory values, arguing against an obvious organic cause.

Recommendations: Given rapid deterioration on Geodon, it is recommended that she continue risperidone. Olanzapine was considered as an alternative since it is also efficacious and leads to less motor and hormonal side effects (prolactin elevation). The family and patient were counseled that the major side effects of olanzapine can be managed behaviorally with diet and exercise. Increasing Prozac was also suggested to provide more aggressive treatment of depressive symptoms. If drug use can be definitively ruled out, and she does not demonstrate further borderline features such as cutting, then it was suggested that clozapine early in treatment would be the most efficacious plan of care. Risks and benefits of clozapine relative to all other agents were discussed with patient and family.

3 ■ Differential Diagnosis: Medical Causes of Psychosis to Distinguish from Schizophrenia

Multiple medical conditions can contribute to or cause psychiatric symptoms. The most prevalent of these disorders are dementias, such as Alzheimer's disease, in which many patients experience hallucinations and delusions. However, onset of mental status changes in these people is during senescence rather than adolescence or early adulthood. Similarly, patients with Huntington's disease may present with a high degree of depressive (approximately 39%) and psychotic symptoms (up to 25%) with a very high suicide rate (Correa, Xavier, & Guimaraes, 2006). However, in this case, there are both a medical cause (axis III) and psychological factors (axis IV). Other conditions ranging form neurosyphilis to neurosarcoidosis can also present with changes in mental status similar to schizophrenia. However, in these cases antibiotics or anti-inflammatory medications are indicated. In the latter case (sarcoidosis with meningeal involvement) the indicated treatment is corticosteroids. However, steroids would likely exacerbate psychosis among people with schizophrenia. Thus, it is critical to make the distinction prior to initiating treatment.

Possible Organic Cause of Psychosis—CASE STUDY 3.1

Source: Patient and mother, review of old records, and consultation with treating psychologist.

History of present illness: The patient is a 23-year-old white male, accompanied by his mother. She is concerned by her son's behavior over the last few years. Specifically, he now has difficulty performing simple vocational tasks such as dishwashing, whereas in high school he had been relatively high functioning. She states he received 1200 on the SAT and average grades, but was recently fired from a job due to inability to arrive on time and wash dishes. Additionally, he made several "concerning" statements regarding odd beliefs of a persecutory nature, accusing her of "switching" sneakers he bought, stating "they didn't feel the same once he got them home," and complaining that someone had come into his room at night and cut his hair. He has become isolated, without close friends and simply "doesn't do anything." The patient states he is not aware of a problem and has no explanation for his inability to work or get to places on time. Until this evaluation he had not thought about his previous abilities relative to his current level of function. He states he has no goals, other than perhaps to "earn $100 per week." He had not considered whether this would meet his financial needs. He cannot elucidate any specifics regarding what he does, why he was present for an evaluation, what his mother is concerned about, or details of his past. He denies poor concentration but has difficulty following the interview.

The patient and his mother state he saw a psychologist 4 years prior for psychological testing, which resulted in a trial of Paxil for several weeks, without noticeable improvement. He discontinued medication against medical advice due to sedation. He also saw a neurologist recently who started him on Ritalin, then a psychiatrist within the past 3 weeks, who discontinued Ritalin and initiated risperidone 0.5 mg per day for "clearer thinking." He received neuropsychological testing again recently but had not received results at the time of evaluation. The patient's mother adds that his friends had "stabbed him in the back" (figuratively) and suspects he'd gotten punched recently after he was "set up in a bad drug deal." The patient states he does not know what the circumstances of his getting punched were. He endorsed occasionally feeling sad and mild anxiety, and he denies sleep or appetite disturbances.

Medical history: Remarkable for a "hairline" fractured skull at 9 months of age with no loss of consciousness.

Medication: Presently receives a prescription for risperidone 1 mg per day (increased after patient's mother spoke with his doctor on the phone to inquire if it would hurt to increase)—the patient states he did not take 5 of the last 6 days worth of medication, but his mother believed he did, at which point he changed his mind.

Social history: He lives in a house with several roommates, but has no close friends. He is working for AmeriCorps at Habitat for Humanity "helping out." He was recently fired from the latest in a series of restaurant jobs for not coming in on time. He states he wakes up early; then doesn't get out in time. He is unable to explain why. Urine toxicology screen was positive for cannabis at recent workup by neurologist. He also states, "I tried LSD once," and occasionally drinks alcohol.

Family history: The patient was raised by his mother after his parents divorced; he has two siblings. History of maternal depression and a paternal grandfather who "died in a mental hospital."

Mental status exam:

Behavior: Uncooperative, guarded, with poor eye contact.

Speech: Remarkable for paucity of content.

Mood: "Fine, why?"

Affect: Angry and irritable.

Thought process: Concrete.

Thought content: Denies suicidal or homicidal ideas, with vague persecutory ideation, responding "not usually," then "I guess never" on further questioning.

Perception: Denies abnormalities.

Insight: Poor: "What do you mean? I'm not having any problem. I'm doing better now than in high school."

Judgment: Poor.

Cognition: Neuropsychological testing 3 months prior indicate a global IQ of 84 with particular difficulties in attention, executive function, and working memory, noting "significant decline in WAIS-R over two assessments." Neuropsychological test 3 years ago indicated full-scale IQ of 98 with performance IQ of 109 with a diagnostic impression at that time of major depression with cluster B personality traits. Neuropsychological testing reveals average to high average function in multiple domains including overall, verbal, and performance IQ; with mild impairments in higher-level problem solving; visual and verbal memory and reaction time; as well as moderate to severe impairments in affect and word recognition.

Laboratories: Liver function tests show mild increase in AST 63 (0–48), otherwise normal; CBC within normal limits; thyroid function tests within normal limits; EEG within normal limits; MRI reveals a smaller cerebellar vermis that his neuroradiologist reads as a normal variant, as well as two areas of increased signal in the periatrial region possibly indicative of a demyelinating process.

Assessment: Patient is a 23-year-old white male who presents for evaluation at the request of his mother. His clinical course has been remarkable for decline in social and occupational function from an average/above average student in high school to average IQ scores in 1995 and is now one standard deviation below the mean (IQ = 85) only 4 years later. His exam is notable for flat affect, avolition, alogia, and vague answers to all questions. He lacks insight into his condition and seems unconcerned with his situation. He endorses mild, positive symptoms including a sense that his things have been switched and someone is entering his room to cut his hair.

1. Presence of two focal abnormalities on MRI is consistent with multiple sclerosis, other demyelinating processes, or Lyme disease. Repeat clinical MRI enhanced with gadolinium may clarify findings.
2. While his presentation is atypical for any one DSM-IV category, one cannot rule out schizophrenia by the following criteria:
   a. Negative symptoms present and delusions possible, although mild.
   b. Social and occupational decline clearly present.
   c. Duration greater than 6 months.
   d. Duration of any affective symptoms have been brief as compared to length of decline in function.
   e. Failure thus far to demonstrate a medical or toxic etiology.
   f. No history of pervasive developmental disorder.

Recommendation: Based on the above criteria, offering empirical treatment with antipsychotic medication is indicated, preferably one with low side effect profile such as olanzapine (10 mg at night). Continue workup of MRI findings to identify potentially treatable etiologies of cognitive decline. Workup should include Lyme titers, RPR, and repeat MRI with enhancement.

■ **Possible Organic Cause of Psychosis**—Case Study 3.2

Sources of information: Patient and his parents.

History of present illness: Patient is a 25-year-old white male who lives with his parents. He was recently admitted to an inpatient psychiatric service. He was transferred from a med/surgery unit due to change in mental status with agitation and psychosis. Upon discharge, it was suggested that he meet with a psychiatrist to obtain a second opinion/clinical consultation regarding both diagnosis and treatment options.

Patient has had hepatic insufficiency (liver problems) since he was a child, which was treated at a children's hospital. The severity of that problem has waxed and waned, with a shunt in place and requiring lactulose for the past 5 years. In the context of existing hepatic insufficiency, he has also had a substantial drinking problem, requiring substance abuse rehabilitation on five occasions by his own report. Both he and his parents note that alcohol greatly exacerbates his behavioral and medical problems. He has been clean for several months by his own account. His behavioral difficulties include becoming very irritable and aggressive. He has had problems with the law, both related to driving while intoxicated and violence while drinking. He lost his driving license and is on probation. He has not been incarcerated. Additionally, he left college with approximately 2 years of credit accrued over the past 5 years. He wishes to return to college and complete his degree. His plan to do so lacks elements of realism in that he plans to go abroad rather than starting locally where family support would be more accessible. His parents support his aspiration to return to school but have a more realistic view of how that might be achieved. Records indicate that the patient has delusions and hallucinations at times. He denies these symptoms and describes ruminative thoughts, may talk to himself to focus, and has been concerned that people wanted to harm him. These experiences do not rise to level of being overtly psychotic or systematized. Records also indicate that he may have had religious delusions, but he and his parents frame this as a normal amount of religious faith, without rising to a pathological symptom. The patient denies frank depression, describing demoralization due to his isolation at home and lack of independence without a driving license or gainful employment. He states he has friends, but does not see them much now because they go out drinking and he cannot join. He does not describe periods of clear mania in the complete absence of substance use and abuse.

Medical history: Hepatic insufficiency since childhood with a shunt, treated with lactulose.

Social history: Alcohol dependence, in remission. He declined to discuss other substances. He lives with his parents, is not presently in a relationship, has friends that he wants to see more than he does, and hopes to resume college soon. He also hopes to resume having a drink each night with dinner, but says he has not acted on that in the past few months. He dismisses the possibility that he may relapse and drink despite being confronted with the observation that he has been drinking for 10 years and has relapsed on every previous quit attempt. As such, he was either unwilling to realistically address the issue with me on our first interaction or truly lacks insight into the severity of the situation.

Psychiatric history: He carries a diagnosis of bipolar disorder, which was made in the context of alcohol abuse and hepatic insufficiency.

Family history: The patient states that no member of his family has had any psychiatric illnesses.

Medications: He states he was previously on lithium, which caused a "severe reaction"; valproate, which caused hepatic difficulties; and risperidone, which was changed during prior admission. He is currently prescribed fluphenazine 1 mg AM and 3 mg PM, although he decreased this himself upon discharge due to a subjective sense of sedation. He also takes lactulose daily.

Mental status exam:

Behavior: Pleasant and cooperative after an initial period of sarcasm and mild verbal antagonism reminiscent of a rebellious teen. This likely reflected not wanting to be here and frustration at being brought to yet another doctor for the same problem he has had for many years. This behavior was nonpathological, and he soon settled into a more appropriate and calm interaction. He did however display a low frustration tolerance, was easily upset by issues he did not want to address, and there were multiple instances that required active redirection to deescalate his affect.

Speech: Normal rate, rhythm, latency of response, and prosody.

Mood: He denies depressed mood, describing periods of demoralization.

Affect: He was bright and joking, which could come off as a cross between a young teenlike demeanor and slightly aggressive sarcasm. He was able to control that and act more appropriately.

Thought process: He was logical and goal directed.

Thought content: Denies frank delusions or aggressive thoughts, no suicidal or homicidal thoughts. He has some resentment about having to live under his parents' rules, consistent with normal adult development in the context of an adult child living at home.

Perception: No hallucinations.

Insight and judgment: Limited appreciation for the likelihood that he will relapse and use alcohol. This is particularly distressing in that his doing so would continue to obscure both his psychiatric diagnosis and his medical and psychiatric prognosis. He has made some very poor choices in the past, especially with respect to alcohol in the context of liver disease. These decisions have been so deleterious that it has raised the issue of where to draw the distinction between simple poor judgment, as seen in substance abuse and addiction, and bona fide psychiatric illness such as bipolar disorder.

Cognition: Concentration and attention appeared fair; memory was grossly intact, formal neuropsychological testing was not performed.

Assessment: The patient is a 25-year-old male seen for diagnostic second opinion and treatment recommendations. He has a lifelong history of hepatic insufficiency that has been exacerbated by alcohol dependence and recurrent abuse. His alcohol problem complicates his psychiatric diagnosis in two major domains.

First, alcohol dependence can often lead to severe and debilitating behavioral problems including many of the symptoms he displays. These include periods of antisocial violent outbursts, driving while intoxicated, arrests, and failure to complete schooling and/or maintain gainful employment. It is difficult, if not impossible, to make a comorbid psychiatric diagnosis during periods of concurrent substance abuse due to the overlapping nature of the behavioral abnormalities. The only way to disentangle the contribution of alcohol from those that are independent of the acute effects of intoxication and protracted effects of dependence is to refrain from substance abuse for a period of 6 months or more. He is at that juncture where his clean time is beginning to accumulate to the point that he could assess a baseline level of function that is not obscured by substance abuse. His ability to remain clean over the next 2–3 months will therefore be the key to clarify his long-term prognosis and plan.

The second complication is that alcohol will exaggerate his underlying hepatic insufficiency to the point that he will become intermittently confused, disoriented, and delirious from the effects of hepatic failure. Thus, he has had two major reasons to display a variety of psychiatric symptoms due to the direct or indirect effects of alcohol on his brain and/or liver. Again, the only way to address this issue will be to refrain from hepatotoxic substances. Unfortunately, virtually all medications are metabolized by the liver, so there will be a period during which he cannot fully refrain from some degree of stress on his liver.

The medications he is currently taking are quite reasonable. Fluphenazine is a good antipsychotic medication that was initiated due to emergent behavioral outbursts. Therefore, its use is justified by the degree of aggression, disorientation, and disability he was experiencing.

Diagnosis: The patient carries a previous diagnosis of bipolar disorder. One function of this consult was to rule out alternative, more severe disorders including schizophrenia that could account for the extent of his disability. He does not have schizophrenia as evidenced by a lack of frank hallucinations, bizarre delusions, negative symptoms, or the occurrence of his disability in the absence of concurrent substance abuse and medical illness.

The main justification for bipolar disorder would be to invoke a diagnosis as a name for the poor judgment that led to substance use (primarily alcohol) in the face of existing liver failure. However, many people exercise poor judgment without having any illness to account for it. This is especially true when those decisions are made as an adolescent as is the case for this individual. It is more likely that he experienced the effects from a confluence of related factors, each of which contributes to his level of dysfunction and disability. His liver and brain will do best if he never uses alcohol again. He does not appear ready to understand or accept that recommendation based on his comments and stated desire to drink in the future. His family inquired about the possibility of liver transplant. He is not presently a candidate for that procedure due to the possibility that his own liver would function adequately in the absence of repeated toxic insult (alcohol and medication). Additionally, there is a poor likelihood that he would be a candidate for an unrelated donor liver given his relatively good state of health. Although a family member could donate a lobe to make a liver available, the risks to both donor and recipient are not justified relative to the level of benefit that could be achieved. A hepatologist or gastroenterologist could confirm or refute this evaluation based on more extensive knowledge of the relative benefits and risks of that procedure in this context. In summary, the concurrent use of alcohol and medication over the past 8–10 years obscures the ability to truly know what his level of function could have been and, importantly, could be in the future.

Recommendations: Fluphenazine is as good as many antipsychotic medications for emergent behavioral control. With the exception of clozapine, nothing is significantly better, so this remains a reasonable choice for temporary behavioral control. If he had bipolar disorder (and I'm not at all certain that he does), then lithium would be the drug of choice given its superior efficacy for everything else in that illness and because it is cleared by the kidneys rather than the liver. However, I would not recommend initiating any new medications at this point. Rather, I would recommend a 1-year plan that, if followed, would clarify the contribution of various factors and help plot a life course:

1. Refrain from alcohol and other substance abuse. Failure to do so will continue to complicate diagnosis and lead to continued medication and toxicity to an already frail hepatic system.
2. Remain on current medications for 6 months and resist the temptation to change things if they are going well. Productive reintegration into society will be important.
3. Take one class at a local community college to reintegrate into a normal functional role; family support and appropriate milestones will be the key to success.
4. After 6 months of being free of symptoms, reduce one medication very slowly such that each small incremental change is observed for at least 1 month before making any additional changes. For example, one could reduce fluphenazine by 1 mg each month over a 3-month period. It will be critical to inform his family and empower them to report any deterioration at the first sign of change. Because this would ideally occur on a backdrop of being free of symptoms for 6 months, any symptoms would be a red flag to resume prior dose.
5. After fluphenazine is discontinued (9 months from now if all goes well), his hepatologist will be in a better position to reassess the

state of the patient's liver in the absence of alcohol and/or medications that are hepatically metabolized.

6. After 3 months off all medication and substances, he will be able to evaluate his true capabilities.

Although this plan sounds simplistic, the sad reality is that most substance abusers do not take the simple steps to stop their self-destructive behaviors. Because of that, they ultimately cause substance-induced medical problems to multiple organ systems including brain and liver. I believe that the patient is not yet beyond the point of no return. However, each recurrence moves him one step closer to a life lost to alcohol. Given his existing hepatic insufficiency, this is truer for him than most other people.

Medical Diagnoses

Dementias

Although psychosis is a prominent component of several dementias, age of onset distinguishes the conditions. This cross-sectional similarity led to the initial designation of dementia precox for schizophrenia due to the recognition that some patients experienced an early form of dementia. Despite the differences in neuropathology and age of onset, both the early dementia (e.g., schizophrenia) and late dementias (e.g., Alzheimer's disease) are treated with similar agents, suggesting some similarity in the mechanisms of psychosis. Alternatively, these agents have no efficacy for the cognitive component of either illness, suggesting that the mechanisms of psychosis and cognitive decline are independent.

Seizure Disorders

Psychosis is not a common presentation in seizure disorders. However, there are forms of seizure disorder that can progress to psychosis. One example of this is called forced normalization seizures. In this form of seizure disorder, patients experience increasingly odd behavior between seizures. In fact, family members say that they can predict when seizures are "due" based on the patient's behavior leading up to an event. Anecdotally, following the typical tonic-clonic generalized seizure, the patient's behavior is "normalized" until they repeat the cycle. Approximately 1% of people with temporal lobe epilepsies develop schizophrenia-like symptoms with frank delusions and hallucinations. The phenomenon of forced normalization also refers to the observation that the seizures "normalize the inter-ictal episodes." The following patient vignette illustrates the interactions between seizure disorders, their treatment, and psychotic episodes.

Seizure Disorder with Concomitant Psychosis— Patient Vignette

The patient presented to the psychiatric service as a 25-year-old male admitted to the inpatient epilepsy monitoring unit. He had a lifelong history of intractable seizures, eventually leading to the placement of an intrathalamic stimulator for seizure control. Shortly after the device had been increased in both frequency and intensity of stimulation, he experienced auditory hallucinations of God talking to him through his teeth, as well as delusions that a woman featured in an online pornographic site was contacting him and sending messages that she and he "were meant to be together." He also displayed bizarre behavior, hiding behind a chair in the hospital and stating that a man was in his room. He became confrontational at home, based on his beliefs that he had to go out at all hours of the night, or leave the front door open so his imaginary lover could find him. He was initially started on antipsychotic medication with moderate treatment response for his psychotic behaviors, experiences, and beliefs. His stimulator was tapered, and eventually discontinued due to the possibility that it contributed to his psychosis. The dose of antipsychotic medication was tapered over 6 months to determine if his symptoms resolved in the absence of his thalamic stimulator. Despite early promise, his psychotic symptoms flared as his antipsychotic medication was decreased. He resumed moderate doses of antipsychotic medication despite removal of the stimulator but has never resumed his previous level of function and can no longer live independently or retain a job. Therefore, his presentation is most consistent with forced normalization. The series of events leading up to his initial presentation likely reflect a progression of his seizure disorder.

Tertiary Syphilis

Rarely, patients present with schizophrenia-like psychosis in the presence of a rash and motor abnormalities including paresis. This may reflect a stage of neurosyphilis, with infection of the central nervous system. In such cases, treating the underlying infection can be curative. It is therefore routine to check a rapid plasma regain (RPR) test to rule out neurosyphilis in all new onset psychosis patients.

Sarcoidosis

Neurosarcoidosis can also present with mental status changes and refractory psychosis (Bona, Fackler, Fendley, & Nemeroff, 1998). In such incidences, there are generally additional signs of sarcoidosis present, including granulomas and skin changes. Although the presentation can be indistinguishable from schizophrenia, the indicated treatments differ. If a diagnosis of sarcoidosis is confirmed, especially in the presence of meningeal inflammation, high-dose steroids are indicated and can resolve the psychotic symptoms. If, however, the patient has schizophrenia, with comorbid sarcoidosis, then steroids may exacerbate the psychotic component. It is important to obtain an MRI to determine if there is evidence of CNS involvement prior to administration of steroids. In such cases, it is prudent to perform the trial of steroids in a highly monitored environment since the outcome can get better, worse, or remain the same.

Traumatic Brain Injury (TBI)

The diagnosis of schizophrenia is often made in the context of previous life events that appear to be contributory to the change in behavior. Often, an incidental life stressor or previous drug abuse can obscure diagnostic clarity. However, a history of previous head trauma can also complicate the diagnostic certainty. Next, we describe two examples of patients with psychosis and history of head trauma.

Psychosis with Incidental Finding of MRI Changes and Possible History of Remote TBI—Clinical Vignette

The patient presented at 18 years of age with auditory hallucinations, paranoid ideation, and confusion. He had previously functioned well in high school and planned to attend college the following year. During his initial inpatient stay, he began clozapine, which was titrated up to a clinically appropriate dose over the ensuing 2 months. The workup for new onset psychosis included an MRI, which revealed a region of hyperintensity in the right frontal pole. When presented with this information, he reported that he was dropped as a baby and hit his head. Details of the incident were vague. He was then diagnosed with traumatic injury-induced psychosis. He displayed dramatic improvement on clozapine over the next years, eventually completing a vocational training program. The delay from the identified incident of injury and onset of psychosis with loss of previously attained level of function suggest he has schizophrenia with incidental MRI changes and possible remote history of trauma that is likely not contributory.

Psychosis with History of Motor Vehicle Accident— Clinical Vignette

The patient initiated care at 25 years of age, when she was admitted to an acute inpatient psychiatric unit. At that time, her family described that she was "normal" until she was a passenger in a motor vehicle accident. Over the ensuing 10 years, she experienced periods of relative health, interspersed with exacerbations and reduced vocational function. Her sibling later developed similar symptoms, suggesting a familial vulnerability to psychosis. Upon further inquiry, her father notes that the patient was always very gregarious and energetic prior to her accident, describing periods that approach manic proportions. Despite an enduring diagnosis of traumatic brain injury-induced change in mental status, the constellation of genetic and premorbid factors suggest the development of a primary psychiatric disorder with an incidental accident.

Surgical (Postsurgical)

Postsurgical patients often become psychotic due to either medical causes of delirium or exposure to anesthetic and analgesic medications. Although the cross-sectional presentation of postsurgical psychosis can be similar to schizophrenia, the root causes and functional significance are distinct. Interestingly, the treatment of postsurgical psychosis is identical to that for psychosis from schizophrenia, namely antipsychotic medications. The major distinction is that postsurgical psychosis will often resolve on its own or upon identification of the causal problem.

4 ■ Etiology and Progression of Illness

Pathophysiology

Approximately 1 out of every 100 people develops schizophrenia. Unlike many psychiatric disorders that are defined by cultural norms, the incidence and expression of schizophrenia is remarkably constant throughout the world and across time. This observation led schizophrenia to be among the first psychiatric disorders to be recognized as a neurological or brain disorder. Although the distinction between a brain disorder and psychological disorder seems antiquated today, most psychiatric disorders were not recognized as having concrete biological substrates until the last quarter century.

Risk Factors

Genetic Vulnerability

Approximately 50% of the risk for schizophrenia can be ascribed to genetic factors. This assertion comes from family and adoption studies that show the risk for schizophrenia is proportional to an individual's biological relationship to an affected patient. For example, there is a 1% prevalence for the disorder in the general population. This risk is increased 10-fold if one has a single first-degree relative that is already diagnosed. For example, the risk for developing schizophrenia is 10% if either parent or a sibling is affected. There is no additional risk conferred if that sibling is a dizygotic twin. However, if a monozygotic twin develops the illness, the relative risk is 50-fold, suggesting fully half of the risk is conferred by sharing the same genome. Similarly, there is a 50% risk of developing schizophrenia if both parents are affected, again supporting the idea that receiving 100% of your genetic material from affected individuals results in 50% risk of illness. There is a proportional dilution effect such that nieces, nephews, and grandchildren of affected patients have approximately 2% to 5% risk, again reflecting approximately one quarter to one half of the risk of a first-degree relation (Figure 4.1) (Gottesman, 1991).

Despite this consistent evidence that genes contribute to the vulnerability to schizophrenia, identifying specific genes that confer risk has been more elusive. A variety of genes have been linked to increased risk, but few are replicated in independent samples, and none account for more than a minimal increase in risk relative to other alleles (O'Tuathaigh et al., 2006). A recent review by Prathikanti and Weinberger (2005) provides an overview of this topic in more detail. Several candidate genes and pathways have been implicated, but much needs to be done to validate and replicate these findings before definitive statements can be made regarding specific genetic risks.

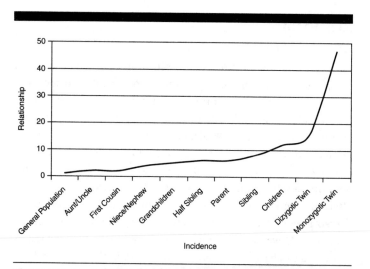

■ **Figure 4.1** Incidence of schizophrenia by genetic proximity.

The incidence of schizophrenia varies in proportion to the degree of genetic similarity with an affected individual. For example, the relative risk for developing the disorder increases 2-fold for first cousins and for uncles and aunts, 5-fold for grandchildren, 10-fold for siblings and other first-degree relatives, and 50-fold for monozygotic twins. Data from Gottesman 1991.

Environmental Factors

A variety of environmental factors have also been shown to add minimal to modest increased risk for schizophrenia. Among these factors, most have yielded mixed results across studies, again suggesting that no one factor reliably increases risk. For example, several studies have suggested that prenatal infections may increase risk (Battle, Martin, Dorfman, & Miller, 1999). These studies generally rely on very slight increase in the prevalence of the disease among offspring that were born following an influenza epidemic. However, approximately as many studies fail to find this association (Cooper, 1992; Crow & Done, 1992; Kendell & Kemp, 1989; Sham et al., 1992). Similarly, prenatal stress has been suggested as a risk for schizophrenia. These studies include increased prevalence among people born during war or if there is a death of the father during gestation (Huttunen & Niskanen, 1978; Myhrman, Rantakallio, Isohanni, Jones, & Partanen, 1996; van Os & Selten, 1998; Yaktin & Labban, 1992). Prenatal nutrition and length of gestation have also been implicated as risks, as evidenced by isolated findings of increased incidence among children born during famine or with premature births (Boog, 2004; Smits, Pedersen, Mortensen, & van Os, 2004). Some of these factors can be traced to an individual (premature birth, death of the father during gestation), but most cases cannot (famine, influenza epidemic, war). This hinders the ability to link specific cases with identifiable risk exposure. Other environmental factors that increase risk include being born in winter months or in an urban setting (Freeman, 1994).

Developmental History

ADHD

Relative Risk of Developing Schizophrenia with a Diagnosis of ADHD

There is a high degree of overlap between the symptoms of attention deficit disorder (ADD) and the earliest signs of schizophrenia. For example, patients early in the process of developing schizophrenia often display problems with memory, attention, and verbal learning. There are many potential causes for these problems, especially among teenagers experiencing a high degree of anxiety during the maturation period around puberty. Many teenagers are given prescriptions for stimulants to aid in their cognitive and behavioral problems. Such interventions are generally helpful regarding motivation and increasing focus in individuals regardless of whether or not there is a bona fide illness. That is to say, low-dose amphetamines will generally prove beneficial for concentration among individuals with or without ADD. However, some people develop mild psychotic symptoms on stimulants (Srisurapanont, Kittiratanapaiboon, & Jarusuraisin, 2001). This further complicates the diagnostic uncertainty between ADD with psychosis secondary to amphetamine use and early so called prodromal schizophrenia (Bellak, Kay, & Opler, 1987).

Relative Risk of Developing Schizophrenia from Treatment with Stimulants

The majority of children diagnosed with ADD do not go on to develop schizophrenia. However, a small subset of these children are actually beginning to exhibit early cognitive signs of a much more serious disease for which amphetamines and other stimulants do not have beneficial effect (Erlenmeyer-Kimling et al., 2000). Quite the contrary, amphetamines may exacerbate or hasten the progression to psychosis among vulnerable patients that have started the inevitable progression to schizophrenia. Despite this propensity to increase psychotic symptoms, there has been very little research regarding the long-term consequences of widespread prescription of amphetamines during adolescence. Thus, the potentially causal links between amphetamine use and later psychosis are unknown.

■ **Possible Stimulant-Induced Psychosis**—Case Study 4.1

Source: Patient along with his mother and father. In addition, records were obtained and reviewed prior to the interview.

Developmental history: Patient was born with forceps according to his parents' report, which they note resulted in birth trauma and developmental difficulties. He was in special education, spoke late, and has an articulation disorder. He was diagnosed with ADHD at a young age, treated with methylphenidate (Ritalin) initially and later amphetamine (Adderall). He completed special education through high school and later completed college for special needs individuals.

History of present illness: The patient is a 24-year-old single male with developmental disabilities. He states he began hearing voices around 19 years of age, while being treated with stimulants for attentional problems. He initially noted some low-level paranoia at that time, with a vague sense that some people may have been trying to harm him. He also notes that he has had periods of sadness and crying that predate the emergence of psychotic symptoms. Records from his treating psychiatrist are consistent with the patient's recollection of events and note that auditory hallucinations were controlled with the addition of aripiprazole (Abilify). His parents note that he has never been treated with other antipsychotic medications. They also note that his attentional problems as a child were profound, impaired his ability to function in school, and were dramatically improved on stimulants. There is no acute change or emergency at the present time.

They note that they attended a recent educational conference and wanted additional information regarding diagnosis and treatment options for their son. The patient lacks a unitary diagnosis for his psychiatric and learning disabilities. His mother notes that they have heard the term *schizophrenia* and are aware that his onset of symptoms is consistent with the usual age of onset for that illness. His parents note that he has been on higher doses of medication at times and developed increased motor difficulties consistent with torticollis while on a very high dose of aripiprazole. He started benztropine (Cogentin) at that time with resolution of stiffness.

The family stated that he has periods of impulsive spending in response to questions directed at bipolar symptoms. However, the pattern of impulsivity and spending is limited to buying music CDs with a portion of his paycheck instead of paying rent to his parents. The patient stated that he resents paying rent, especially since he has so little money and his parents have plenty. Despite a brief conversation regarding the possibility that the rent is part of his parents' desire to teach him responsible life strategies to manage his money, the patient does not agree with or like this logic. His spending appeared more as a way to protest his need to pay rent than any true psychiatric symptom.

Medical history: The patient has no other medical conditions. Records indicate he had jaw surgery when younger.

Social history: He lives with his parents, has few friends, and works part-time at a supermarket. He wants to work more. His parents say they had anticipated that he would be able to hold a higher-level job than he currently has, potentially working with computers. He does not have a girlfriend but has interest in dating. He has never used illicit drugs or alcohol.

Medication: Aripiprazole 30 mg (as high as 45 mg in past), Adderall 30 mg recently decreased from 40 mg, Cogentin 2 mg/day and escitalopram (Lexapro) 20 mg/day.

Family history: Paternal aunt died while in a psychiatric facility. The patient has a brother with ADD, who is treated effectively with atomoxitine (Strattera). The patient has two other brothers with no known psychiatric difficulties.

Mental status exam:

Appearance: Dressed neatly in normal clothes appropriate to his age.
Behavior: Pleasant and cooperative.
Speech: Dysarthric, due to primary articulation disorder that predates treatment with antipsychotic medication.
Mood: "OK," although he notes he is sometimes sad and cries, even when he cannot identify a reason.
Affect: Restricted but appropriate.
Thought process: Logical in flow.

Thought content: No suicidal, homicidal, or aggressive ideation; no delusions.

Perception: None currently; history of auditory hallucinations that occur approximately 1 time per week.

Insight: Good, he understands his situation and is unhappy with how things have turned out. Some of his demoralization and behavior is likely due to the difficult nature of his situation.

Judgment: Fair, at times he indulges his desire to rebel against his parents' rules. However, this is likely a way to vent his frustration at his entire life situation rather than a symptom.

Impulse control: Situationally poor, not likely true impulse control disorder, more likely frustration-based choices.

Cognition: Although he matriculated through special education, he had no difficulty following the interview or making his opinions clearly understood by others. IQ appears to be within normal range.

Assessment: Patient is a 24-year-old male with developmental disabilities likely related to birth trauma. His attentional problems were well controlled with stimulants as a child. He later developed limited psychotic symptoms while being treated with stimulants, raising the possibility that his hallucinations were medication-induced rather than idiopathic. At that time he was treated with aripiprazole, which itself can have stimulant-like properties when used at doses above 15 mg. Of note, the initial published clinical trials with this mediation showed better efficacy at 15 mg than higher doses. It is common, however, for physicians to increase the dose based on algorithms developed with other medications (e.g., if low dose does not work, then increase). That may not be effective for aripiprazole due to its partial agonist properties. It is therefore possible that the combination of stimulants (Adderall) and a stimulating dose of aripiprazole are now contributing to his psychosis. Using Cogentin as an antidote for aripiprazole is unusual. Since aripiprazole is a partial agonist at dopamine receptors, the strategy of countering its effects with anticholinergic medication is not clear. The Lexapro seems appropriate for his depressive symptoms, although his report is also consistent with emotional incontinence, which could be resistant to antidepressant medications.

Recommendations: Since there is a high likelihood that he is experiencing stimulant-induced hallucinations, I recommend tapering the Adderall. However, the aripiprazole could also be exacerbating the situation. I suggest that any number of older and also effective medications would be appropriate if he has psychotic symptoms after his stimulant is reduced or discontinued. Cogentin is not necessarily indicated and should be stopped as soon as his other medications are at lower doses.

Changes should be slow and metered with involvement of the family and close observation at weekly or biweekly intervals throughout the change.

I suggest first lowering the Adderall by 10 mg/month to a dose that is less likely to contribute to psychosis. He may be able to stop it now that he is older.

I would then suggest lowering aripiprazole by 10 mg/month until it is discontinued. A maximum of 10–15 mg may be tolerated, albeit there may be alternate medications available to counter Adderall-induced psychosis.

Cogentin could be lowered by 1 mg/week and used only as needed until he is weaned from aripiprazole and Adderall. He should not be on standing anticholinergic medications, as these are likely to contribute to cognitive problems and are not indicated at the much lower doses of his other medications.

If he resumes having profound attentional and behavioral problems once off the Adderall, he could resume low doses (e.g., 10–15 mg/day) with slow titration to the lowest effective dose.

If he experiences medication-induced hallucinations at that time, I suggest using a more conventional antipsychotic medication that does not have the potential to mimic amphetamine. Olanzapine, risperidone, or perphenazine are good choices. There are other medications that one could use as well.

Mild Mental Retardation vs. Cognitive Impairment of Schizophrenia—CASE STUDY 4.2

Source: The patient is a 22-year-old Asian male college student who reports trouble concentrating on school work. Information was obtained from his mother, referring counselor, and prior psychiatrist, as well as school records.

History of present illness: The patient describes difficulty completing assignments at school, with difficulty comprehending and concentrating. He is very anxious about work and his desire to "get an education." He describes a great deal of difficulty throughout his educational career, with last "good" performance in "3rd grade." He went to summer school to complete high school. Records indicate he finished 568th of 601 in his class with a combined SAT score of 530/1600 (230 verbal, 300 math). Additionally, he had difficulty at junior college. He first engaged in counseling at that time secondary to his academic performance. He is now at an art institute, where he experienced difficulties and has seen a school counselor for the past year. His counselor reports he has become increasingly anxious and more confused. Additionally, the counselor became concerned the patient might be hearing voices, although the specifics are vague: the patient cannot describe whether he hears people in the adjacent room or voices of people who are not present. Upon further questioning, the patient reports hearing only his name in crowded places (which is considered a normal experience). There is no evidence of true auditory hallucinations. Additionally, there has been concern regarding persecutory ideation. Again, the patient is extremely vague and appears highly suggestible, stating only, "I don't know why anyone would try to hurt me, but other guys make fun of me sometimes, especially when they drink alcohol at parties."

Past medical history: None.

Psychiatric history: Saw a psychiatrist at counselor's recommendation approximately 3 months prior for "trouble with work."

Medication: None.

Mental status exam:

Behavior: Pleasant, 22-year-old male appearing his stated age with mild restlessness.

Speech: Mild slowing.

Mood: "Anxious."

Affect: Full range and appropriate.

Thought process: Logical and goal directed, but simple and at times demonstrating confusion regarding questions.

Thought content: No evidence of suicidal or homicidal ideation, nor any delusional content.

Perception: There is no evidence for perceptual abnormalities.

Insight: Limited.

Judgment: Fair.

Cognitive abilities: Grossly consistent with borderline mental retardation, meaning he could not perform simple arithmetic and had difficulty understanding conversation at times.

Assessment: The patient is a 22-year-old male with long-standing limited cognitive capacity and recent anxiety that renders him unable to fulfill his academic tasks. There is no evidence of psychosis or schizophreniform disorder.

Recommendation: The patient may benefit from consultation with a general psychiatrist for treatment of anxiety. If the patient and family so desire, neuropsychological testing could be performed to determine level of cognitive impairment.

Contribution of Drug Abuse

Schizophrenia vs. Drug Abuse vs. Sociopathy—
CASE STUDY 4.3

Source: Patient was seen in consultation at the request of his family. Records were obtained and reviewed prior to the interview. The patient was interviewed alone initially and then in the presence of his mother.

History of present illness: Patient is a 29-year-old male who describes a long history of problems since 16 years of age, "since the time I had sex with five girls in the science room at school." His report of this incident and its significance has delusional character, in both lack of detail, implausibility, and his statement that he disappeared afterwards and knew it was real because he was "clean and sober before that and still could not remember it." That lack of logic pervaded the interview. He states he then began using drugs, including marijuana, LSD, and ecstasy ("E"), the last of which he states he overdosed with at 19 years of age "for no reason—I just took 10 because my friend was going to sell them." He states he had been in rehab for "all the drugs" prior to his OD incident at age 19. The interview was very strained due to both the patient's disorganization of thought, lack of logical flow, and frank hostility. He noted that he did not go to college. He has worked several jobs over the last 10 years. He liked landscaping best but frequently got in fights with other workers. He stated that he twice assaulted a friend with whom he does drugs, resulting in a 3-month and subsequent 5-month period in jail. When asked how he felt about having assaulted this friend, he stated, "I hope I broke his skull" in a matter of fact tone, but could not clarify why he said that. He initially stated that he has been clean and sober since he was incarcerated 8 months ago, then added, "Actually I did crack cocaine and marijuana last weekend."

The patient states he has "heard voices," but then tried to recant that statement, saying that it was actually people in the neighborhood messing with his thoughts and controlling him. He lacked insight to realize that the latter explanation was not "normal" either. He contradicted himself repeatedly, often in the context of saying that "It's a defense mechanism" despite the inability to explain what that psychiatric jargon meant. He's been treated with risperidone, lithium, ziprasidone (Geodon), and valproic acid (Depakote) in the past, but was not able to provide any sense of his diagnoses. He stated only, "Now my mother is saying schizophrenia, which really pisses me off." He stated that he had no symptoms in prison, but appeared to be such a poor historian that it is impossible to interpret the significance of that report.

The interview ended abruptly when he said, "Jews make my eyes have spots. It's because I believe in Hitler." When confronted that saying such things was inappropriate and aggressive, he became very agitated and appeared to be on the verge of violence. At that juncture, he was told to leave the room and bring his mother in to wrap up and finish. During the final portion with his mother he was argumentative and verbally provocative, attempting to get the psychiatrist into a confrontation.

Developmental history: He did not describe any developmental disorders or difficulties in school prior to the episode at 16 and subsequent drug use. He has a GED.

Medical history: Obesity.

Social history: He lives with his parents, has no friends, and states that all of his problems stem from his inability to interact with women. He made several illusions to not being gay. He denied homosexual relationships or feelings previously or presently. He also used the phrase "that guy thought he had dibs on me" suggesting he may have been the property of another inmate while incarcerated. He denied that he was referring to prison. He does not work. He has used drugs extensively including crack, marijuana, LSD, and ecstasy. He may have inhaled solvents in high school according to collateral reports.

Medication: Currently taking risperidone 1 mg AM and 2 mg PM as well as Depakote ER 250 mg AM and 500 mg PM (he may have reported wrong pill strength—given how low the resulting dose would be, it is possible it is actually twice that if he has 500 mg tablets). He states he was on Geodon previously, which he preferred. It is less clear that it worked well for him given his incarceration and lack of impulse control.

Mental status exam:

Appearance: Poor attention to personal appearance and hygiene, picking at a lesion on his face throughout the interview.

Behavior: Aggressive, staring at me while making provocative comments.

Speech: Normal rate, rhythm, and volume with long latency of response.

Mood: "OK."

Affect: Flat through most of the interview. However, he became animated and aggressive toward the end, staring intensely in apparent effort to appear menacing.

Thought process: Moderate thought disorder, creating a very strained interview due to inability to keep him on topic or to follow logical stream of his answers.

Thought content: No suicidal or homicidal ideation. He denied that he would hurt his mother on the way home. Delusions present for mind control and accusing me of being part of a conspiracy. Also multiple grandiose delusions, most notably related to his sexual and physical prominence in high school and how "people are still talking about that" and treating him differently due to those (likely imaginary) events.

Perception: No current auditory hallucinations, unclear history due to frequent alteration of his story in the service of trying to deemphasize psychiatric illness.

Insight: Very poor.

JUDGMENT: Very poor.

Impulse control: Very poor.

Cognition: Limited. However, he had one moment of clarity after he demanded to know my credentials. After hearing "4 years of college, 4 years of medical school, 4 years of PhD, 4 years of residency, 2 years of fellowship, and 6 years in practice," he responded immediately with, "then you're over 40," suggesting he was able to process the numbers. Oddly, learning that I was much older than he realized calmed him considerably.

Assessment: Patient is a 29-year-old male with complicated history consistent with either:

1. Psychotic disorder and comorbid substance abuse.
2. Polysubstance-induced psychotic disorder.

3. Antisocial personality disorder and sociopathy leading to violent acts and drug use.

Patient is a poor historian. As noted by the patient, his current medication regimen includes very low doses of medication, less consistent with treating the psychiatric etiology as primary. However, his thought disorder and delusional conviction, coupled with his anger at the intimation he has a psychiatric illness, favor a primary psychiatric etiology. Given his extensive drug use and possible history of using inhalants, it is also possible that his psychiatric symptoms are real, but follow toxic, drug-induced alterations in brain function, leading to a lasting deficit state. Alternatively, the objectionable behaviors, including violence, threats, and the inflammatory pro-Nazi views he espouses do not engender empathy, likely leading people in the criminal justice and medical communities to view him as a sociopath rather than a patient. That may well be the case. However, until adequately treated it is not possible to rule out either a bona fide illness such as schizophrenia/bipolar disorder or a substance-induced toxic psychotic state. Only protracted sobriety (which he has not achieved) will allow one to rule out current substance abuse as contributory.

Recommendations: I suggest more aggressive treatment for his psychotic and impulsive behaviors. If his dose of valproate really is 750 mg/day (he reports 3 × 250), then it is too low to control true bipolar disorder or frontal release impulsivity. This dose could be increased to 25–50 mg/kg/day, which would be 2500–5000 mg/day in his case (100 kg). He could therefore take two 500-mg tabs in AM and three 500-mg tabs before bed for a total of 2500 mg per day and titrate up from there. Similarly, his current dose of risperidone is quite low given his body mass. Although 3 mg/day is adequate for many patients of 60–70 kg, a 100-kg man such as this could easily tolerate 5 or 6 mg, especially given his propensity for violence while in a psychotic state. Therefore, I recommend more aggressive treatment including 2–3 mg of risperidone and 1000 mg of Depakote ER in the AM and 3 mg of risperidone and 1500–2000 mg of Depokote

ER in the PM. These doses could then be adjusted up and/or down based on his progress and side effects. The risks to him, his family, and society of undertreating him outweigh the risks to him of overly sedating him.

Relative Risk from Drugs of Abuse

The relative risk and contribution of premorbid drug abuse toward the development of schizophrenia remains unclear. Several studies suggest that there is increased substance abuse among people who eventually develop schizophrenia (Arias Horcajadas, 2007; Bangalore et al., 2008; Serper, Chou, Allen, Czobor, & Cancro, 1999). Among drugs of abuse, cannabis abuse has been most frequently linked to the later development of schizophrenia. This may reflect a directionally causal relationship between marijuana use during adolescence and later development of schizophrenia. Alternatively, the preponderance of evidence for cannabis as a risk factor may simply reflect the relative frequency of marijuana abuse relative to other drugs. Alternatively, a predisposition to schizophrenia may increase the likelihood of drug abuse during the prodromal period, increasing the apparent correlation. Data linking cocaine to later development of schizophrenia has largely focused on the consequences of prenatal exposure as a relative risk for later behavioral abnormalities. Although there is little evidence for a causal relationship between cocaine use in adulthood and development of schizophrenia, the acute presentation of cocaine toxicity can masquerade as schizophrenia in the emergency room setting. Therefore, the cross-sectional appearance of schizophrenia cannot be assessed without a toxicological screen to rule out drugs of abuse. A diagnosis of schizophrenia cannot be made during or directly following a period of intoxication. This is especially true for a subset of drugs including phencyclidine (PCP), ketamine (Special K), nitrous oxide, and other so-called "club drugs" such as MDMA (Ecstasy) that can lead to protracted psychotic symptoms, negativistic behaviors, and cognitive deficits lasting up to 1 week in some cases. There are some clear neurotoxins that can be used as drugs of abuse, leading to lasting changes in brain function and behavior. These include inhaling or "huffing" gasoline and formaldehyde. Thus, a comprehensive drug history can help elucidate correlative factors that may contribute to the presentation of schizophrenia.

Schizophrenia affects behavior, perception, and cognition with resulting impairments in multiple functional domains. The severity and chronicity of schizophrenia has stimulated examination of sociodemographic and clinical variables at presentation as predictors of outcome. While this has yielded several consistent conclusions, inconsistencies are also apparent. Several studies suggest that illness course differs between men and women (Hambrecht, Maurer, Hafner, & Sartorius, 1992; Loebel et al., 1992; Szymanski et al., 1995), while others do not (Browne et al., 2000; Ho, Andreasen, Flaum, Nopoulos, & Miller, 2000; Kendler & Walsh, 1995). Because similar measures may have different predictive values depending on stage of illness, some inconsistencies between different studies may relate to samples that mixed new-onset and chronic patients.

The study of first-episode patients has received increased attention in neurobiology (McGlashan, 1999; Thakore, 2004) and treatment research (Lieberman et al., 1996; Wyatt, Damiani, & Henter, 1998). Yet, few studies examine differences in prognostic factors between first episode and previously treated patients (Lieberman et al., 1992; Szymanski, Cannon, Gallacher, Erwin, & Gur, 1996). These studies found similarities and differences between these groups in presentation and outcome. Earlier studies indicated that first-episode and previously treated patients improve in positive symptoms at 6-month, 1-year, and 2-year follow-up, while only previously treated patients show a reduction in negative symptoms (Eaton, Thara, Federman, & Tien, 1998; Gupta et al., 1997; Szymanski et al., 1996). It is unclear whether the reduction in negative symptoms for previously treated patients reflects a later stage of illness or if negative symptoms were less prominent at onset in first-episode patients. This highlights the value of evaluating stage of illness when assessing the prognostic significance of symptoms and other predictors.

Some studies report that symptom severity at intake correlates with symptom-based and quality-of-life outcomes in first-episode patients (Browne et al., 2000; Robinson et al., 1999), yet others fail to find such correlations (Lastra et al., 2000). For example, positive symptom severity at intake is correlated with poor outcome at 1-year (Robinson et al., 1999), and better long-term outcome (23 years) but not 2–8 years (Jonsson & Nyman, 1984). Negative symptoms have also been assessed in first-episode patients with mixed results such that they are correlated with poor functioning at intake and 2 years (Addington, McCleary, & Munroe-Blum, 1998) but not 1-year follow-up (Robinson et al., 1999).

A 5-year study found depressive symptoms in 75% of first-episode patients at intake using the Hamilton Depression Scale (HAMD) (Koreen et al., 1993). Furthermore, depressive symptoms were correlated with both positive and negative symptoms and resolved as psychotic symptoms resolved (Koreen et al., 1993). However, studies examining the significance of depressive symptoms in first-episode patients have yielded mixed results. Depressive symptoms were poorly correlated with 1-year outcome in one study (Robinson et al., 1999), but others concluded that depressive symptoms predict early remission while flat affect predicts longer episodes and shorter remissions (Eaton et al., 1998).

Thus, there are inconsistencies in outcome studies investigating the role of sex, age, and symptoms, as well as the difference between first-episode and previously treated schizophrenia.

Selectivity to Specific Issues

The issue of capacity to provide informed consent for medical decisions is often raised for patients with schizophrenia. This concern is logical, given that so many patients lack insight into their illness and base important decisions on psychotic content. However, schizophrenia alone does not necessarily remove an individual's capacity. Rather, a capacity evaluation must be limited to specific issues at a specific time. The following clinical vignette highlights the distinction between a situation in which a patient lacked capacity for one medical decision while retaining capacity for others.

Capacity to Provide Informed Consent—Clinical Vignette

The patient is a 45-year-old male with somatic delusions related to his back. He believes that his back became injured at the time of his first psychotic episode. He states he was the strongest man in the world at that time, then went to the emergency room, where the doctors put a probe up his rectum, causing back pain and weakness for the following 20 years. He has constructed an elaborate back brace from garbage he finds on the street to help him heal. Occasionally he asks his psychiatrist to help him put on the brace because he believes that the brace allows him to fly. When he requests surgery and other interventions to fix his back, he lacks capacity to provide informed consent, since these decisions are based entirely on psychotic content. However, this same patient is entirely capable of making appropriate decisions about his antipsychotic medications and other medical conditions such as diabetes and hypertension. Thus, his lack of capacity is circumscribed to a particular medical domain that relates to his particular delusions.

Role of the Family

At times when patients with schizophrenia need to make important medical decisions, it is critical to involve family members. This is true to a greater extent than for unaffected individuals for a variety of reasons. As noted above, many patients lack insight, which may impair their ability to comprehend the risks and benefits of their choices. There are no concrete regulations that require involvement of family on a routine basis for people with schizophrenia, and the physician must always balance the need for autonomy with the health and welfare of the patient. In general, it is the family that will know the context of the patient's decision and will ultimately have to deal with the consequences of those choices. Thus, it becomes both helpful and beneficial to allow them to participate in major medical choices.

Medical

Virtually any medical problem can coexist with schizophrenia. However, there are a few that occur with higher frequency than might be expected as a result of the illness or its treatment. For example, most antipsychotic medications cause moderate to severe weight gain secondary to increased hunger. This increase in caloric intake is exacerbated by the sedentary lifestyle among most patients, leading to a variety of obesity-related conditions. Thus, hypertension and type II diabetes are of particular concern among this population. Additionally, the high incidence of smoking among people with schizophrenia leads to a disproportionate incidence of smoking-related pulmonary diseases and cancer. Poor hygiene, bad eating habits, and isolation from medical care also exacerbate the propensity for many schizophrenia patients to suffer from untreated medical conditions. Often, psychiatrists must therefore assume the primary care role and work diligently to engage patients in appropriate medical care. Several medical conditions can also cause psychosis and masquerade as schizophrenia. Neurological, endocrine, and infectious causes of psychosis are discussed further in Chapter 3 (Differential Diagnosis). Additionally, the impact of schizophrenia on various medical conditions is discussed in greater detail in Chapter 8 (Information for Specialties).

Psychiatric

Schizophrenia with Comorbid Depression

The following clinical vignette illustrates the overlap among the symptoms of depression, demoralization due to adverse life events, and negative symptoms. This overlap can be quite difficult to distinguish but ultimately dictates the appropriate course of treatment and prognosis.

Schizophrenia with Depressive Symptoms—Clinical Vignette

The patient is a 35-year-old woman with a 15-year history of schizophrenia. She has held part-time jobs from time to time, often terminating due to her inability to tolerate the stress of entry-level positions or due to her employer noting her difficulty with social interactions. She is relatively isolated, having few if any friends. Because of all these factors (isolation, lack of activity, and lack of function), she reports feeling depressed. Over the course of treatment, this subjective sense of depressed mood has been related to specific factors in her life such as losing a job, lacking a social life, or living with her parents as an adult. As such, it has usually been interpreted as demoralization (i.e., the loss of morale) rather than a psychiatric symptom. Complicating this interpretation, she also describes lack of motivation and lack of enjoyment. These feelings are consistent with a diagnosis of depression, but they are equally consistent with negative symptoms of schizophrenia (see Chapter 1 for description of negative symptoms of schizophrenia). Thus, three explanations for the subjective report of *depression* lead to three potential courses of action.

It is important to recognize that antidepressants have no efficacy for either demoralization or negative symptoms of schizophrenia (Rummel, Kissling, & Leucht, 2006). In these cases, addition of an antidepressant medication is contraindicated, as it adds risk (side effects and drug interactions with antipsychotic medication) without benefit. Alternatively, antidepressants have clear indication and efficacy for a diagnosis of major depression.

The patient has also described worsening of her depressed mood with crying and thoughts of suicide at times. In these instances, trials of selective serotonin reuptake inhibitors (SSRIs) were attempted. She reacted to these medications poorly, complaining of large side effect burden and worsening psychosis, leading to premature termination of the course of treatment.

Over the course of time, the most copasetic explanation for her report is demoralization, since her mood responds to good events (e.g., a new job, a trip with her family, or any activity she enjoys). The focus of her care is therefore to maintain an antipsychotic medication for positive symptoms (see Chapter 1 for definition of positive symptoms of schizophrenia) and therapies to help her create circumstances that enhance her vocational function and social interactions.

The diagnosis of major depression is most often made by primary care physicians, and most antidepressant medication is most often prescribed in a primary care environment. Therefore, it is critical for primary care physicians to recognize that people with schizophrenia have multiple causes for the apparent signs and symptoms of depression, one of which indicates antidepressant medication (major depression) and others in which these medications are contraindicated. It is therefore prudent to defer treatment of psychiatric conditions in this unique population to their psychiatrist, preferably one that specializes in the treatment of schizophrenia.

Substance Abuse

The term *dual diagnosis* refers to the co-occurrence of substance abuse and a psychiatric illness. In rare cases, it is possible to disentangle the relative contribution of these two factors. However, it is most commonly not possible since psychosis often emerges during adolescence and early adulthood when drug use and abuse are common. Additionally, it is rare that patients give up all substance use throughout the course of their illness. Thus, one is left relying on clinical judgment to decide whether or not there is a true illness in the context of substance abuse or only the intermittent presentation of intoxication and interepisode periods of relative normalcy. Of note, there is increasing evidence that many drugs of abuse result in protracted periods of brain dysfunction across a broad range of cognitive, behavioral, and sensory abnormalities lasting weeks to months after cessation of drug use (Majewski-Tiedeken, Rabin, & Siegel, 2008; Maxwell, Ehrlichman, et al., 2006). The following case study illustrates the difficulty in trying to distinguish drug abuse from mental illness.

Comorbid Alcoholism and Mild Traumatic Brain Injury—
CASE STUDY 4.4

Source: The patient is a 43-year-old male seen for a consultation and diagnostic impression.

History of present illness: He states that all was going well until 16 years of age when "I felt like I was being firebombed by everyone," which he attributes to two uses of LSD and mushrooms. He states a priest molested him. He told his mother 5 years later. The patient's father mentions there was a public scandal with this particular priest, supporting that the events described by the patient predated any psychosis and are not delusional in nature.

The patient notes that he began hearing auditory hallucinations at 16. He entered the hospital at that time. He received a diagnosis of schizophrenia, later returning to school to receive a GED. He states the voices have continued for the last 28 years. He takes his medication, but symptoms persist despite good adherence. He drinks alcohol when he feels bad, which complicates fluctuations in symptoms. Of note, he bangs his head against the walls sufficiently hard that he has band-aids covering the wounds. He does this whenever he "feels bad" and has done so for 25 years.

Psychiatric and medical history: He is currently taking Zyprexa 15 mg, and he took haloperidol in the past with a dystonic reaction. He took Cogentin and fluphenazine (Prolixen) (oral and depot formulations) while incarcerated for public drunkenness more than 20 years ago. He also stole a ring and other "crazy things." He took aripiprazole, which made him feel "cloudy," Geodon, which was, "terrible," and perphenazine (Trilafon), which was "not so good." Of all the medications he has had, alprazolam (Xanax) is his favorite.

Family history: His mother abused alcohol during pregnancy with him. Her alcohol abuse later led to liver failure. The patient has a younger brother with bipolar disorder and three sisters without psychiatric disorders.

Social history: He drinks very heavily, having participated in multiple inpatient and outpatient rehabs, last being 4 years ago. He continues to drink heavily, albeit sporadically. He lives alone and works intermittently, delivering circulars. He is on social security disability to support himself. After a bout of heavy drinking, he tries to obtain Xanax to avoid withdrawal.

Mental status exam:

Appearance: Older than stated age.
Behavior: Cooperative with the exam.
Speech: Normal rate and volume.
Mood: "Up and down."
Affect: Restricted.
Thought process: Organized for much of the discussion with tangents and periods of disorganization. For example, he told a story about a woman and angels and "a will and a way" that was very difficult to follow.
Thought content: He does not express either suicidal or homicidal ideation or thoughts of harm and denies frank delusions presently.
Perception: Describes auditory hallucinations.
Insight: Into his drinking problem.
Judgment: Poor about fixing his drinking problem.

Assessment: The patient is a 43-year-old male with significant alcohol abuse and dependence and has experienced consistent psychosis on medication over the past 26 years. He meets criteria for schizophrenia and alcohol dependence. Additionally, regular, moderately severe head trauma may be contributing to his limitations, especially if these lead to frontal lobe damage based on the type of self-injury he commits.

Recommendations: First and foremost he needs to stop drinking alcohol. Nothing will help ameliorate his symptoms and disability in the face of continued alcohol dependence. Olanzapine (Zyprexa) is a very good medication, albeit 15 mg is not the full therapeutic dose, and he could easily go to 20 mg. Given his lack of response to so many medications (Haldol, Prolixin, Trilafon, Geodon, and Abilify), he could also try Clozaril. However, given how difficult it is to take Clozaril, he is not presently able to take that while so invested in drinking.

In summary, he would do much better, even gain full-time employment and a fuller life, if he committed to stopping alcohol and initiating Clozaril. I discussed the possibility of engaging in another rehabilitation effort with an addiction psychiatrist—we would devise a plan together if the patient is willing to participate in rehabilitation.

5 ▪ Neurobiology of Schizophrenia

Neuropathology

"Schizophrenia is the graveyard of neuropathologists." This quote characterized neuroanatomical studies of schizophrenia for the first half of the 1900s (Harrison, 1999; Plum, 1972). However, this former period of scientific quiescence in psychiatry gave way to the current explosion of biological research, led in part and perhaps best exemplified by schizophrenia research. Initial neuroanatomic findings were limited to the observation of enlarged ventricles in schizophrenia. Although this remains the most consistent and replicable finding in the field, it lacks specificity. Subsequent studies have elucidated some possible mechanisms of this increased ventricle-to-brain ratio (VBR), including smaller neuron size and decreased neuron counts in select brain regions (Harrison, 1999). However, with this explosion of research, the lack of data that characterized the early 1900s has been supplanted by a gross excess of findings without either replication or a coherent sense of how these myriad findings fit together. Thus, today's challenge is no longer to find abnormalities but to separate the proverbial chaff from the wheat and determine which findings are real and which will persevere to form a meaningful piece of the puzzle. Several high-quality reviews have attempted to bring order to small subsets of the data. For example, a review by David Lewis and colleagues argues convincingly that there is a selective decrease in a subset of GABAergic interneurons that express the calcium-binding protein parvalbumin (Lewis, Hashimoto, & Volk, 2005). These cells are notable for sending their axons to the axon initial segment of neocortical pyramidal cells in layer 4, thus having the potential to act as gatekeepers for the cortical output from a specific cortical region or column (Figure 5.1) (Lewis, Volk, & Hashimoto, 2004).

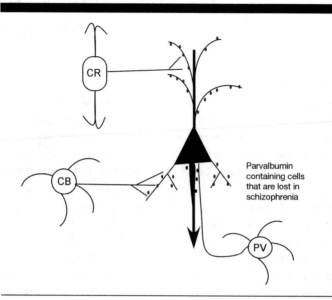

Parvalbumin
containing cells
that are lost in
schizophrenia

■ **Figure 5.1**   **Morphological and biochemical features of subpopu-**
lations of inhibitory cortical GABA (γ-aminobutyric
acid) neurons in the prefrontal cortex.

The diagram illustrates the calcium-binding proteins parvalbumin (PV),
calbindin (CB) and calretinin (CR) and the locations of inhibitory synaptic inputs to a pyramidal neuron (Pyr) by different classes of interneurons. The parvalbumin-containing interneurons provide inhibitory input
to the axon initial segment, shown at the base of the pyramidal cell.
Calbindin- and calretinin-expressing neurons provide inhibitory inputs
to the distal dendrites of pyramidal neurons.

Additionally, this subset of parvalbumin-containing neurons
has the highest proportion of N-methyl-D-aspartate (NMDA)
receptors, relative to other GABAergic cell classes, as defined by
their calcium-binding proteins (Huntley, Vickers, & Morrison,
1997). Thus, there has been a convergence of this line of neu-

roanatomical research with one of the major pharmacological, neurotransmitter-based theories of schizophrenia, namely the NMDA receptor hypofunction theory of schizophrenia. This line of studies has postulated that people with schizophrenia have a reduction in NMDA-type glutamate-mediated transmission. These theories were initially based on the observation that NMDA antagonists such as phencyclidine and ketamine result in behavioral, cognitive, and physiologic profiles similar to those seen in schizophrenia. Subsequent studies have extended this line of research with anatomical studies of NMDA receptors in postmortem brains and genetic studies to examine the genes for proteins involved in the NMDA receptor-mediated signal transduction (Hahn et al., 2006). Among these, the genes for neuregulin-1 and dysbindin have been among the most promising to date (Hahn et al., 2006; Talbot et al., 2004). However, as noted above, genetic studies thus far have only been able to account for very a small amount of the variance for developing schizophrenia, and few have been replicated across populations (Prathikanti & Weinberger, 2005). In this respect, the dysbindin association is perhaps the most consistent. However, mutations in this gene result in muscular dystrophy rather than schizophrenia-like syndromes, complicating interpretation of the genetic findings. Alternatively, functional studies in postmortem brains show increased neuregulin-1 activity in schizophrenia (Hahn et al., 2006). Neuregulin-1 is thought to inhibit NMDA receptor-mediated glutamate transmission (Christ, Wettwer, & Ravens, 2005). Therefore, increased neuregulin-1 activity is among the most promising mechanistic leads for beginning a molecular or mechanistic understanding of schizophrenia.

Behavioral Measures of Schizophrenia

As noted above, medications for schizophrenia have not been substantially changed in over 50 years. This lack of significant change in medication for schizophrenia is in part due to a lack of adequate basic science research tools. One important mechanism to identify new medicines is through the use of animal models. Appropriate animal models of schizophrenia would require a solid understanding of the biological abnormalities that lead to impaired behaviors or function. In such a case, one could create the relevant biological change with drugs, lesions, or gene manipulations prior to measuring an appropriate behavioral change. Unfortunately, clear biological targets and mechanisms do not yet exist for schizophrenia. There are several candidate models that have been used. For example, there is substantial evidence that alterations in the neurotransmitter dopamine are involved in both the biology of schizophrenia and its treatment (reviewed above). Therefore, several animal models incorporate ways to increase dopamine in the brains of an animal. These include drugs that cause increased dopamine release, like amphetamine, as well as those that mimic dopamine directly, like apomorphine. After giving these drugs, several behaviors become abnormal in experimental animals. The second element that is required for an animal model is a measurable behavior or physiological outcome. Ideally these measures also bear some resemblance to the impairments in schizophrenia.

However, the most prominent abnormalities in schizophrenia are hallucinations, delusions, disorganized thought, and impaired judgment. Unfortunately, none of these are possible to measure in experimental animals. Therefore, surrogate markers for these abnormalities have been developed based on the concepts of either face validity or construct validity to the illness. Face validity refers to a behavior or measure that looks similar between species. For example, if a drug causes an animal to stand still, it has face validity for the property of causing stiffness and immobility in humans. Construct validity refers to the idea that you are measuring the same process or idea in both species. For example, a drug that causes animals to perform poorly on a memory task, like remembering where they found food, might have construct validity for memory impairments in schizophrenia. Predictive validity is a third concept used in treatment development. Predictive validity refers to the extent to which the effect of a drug in animals accurately predicts some known effect in people. For example, amphetamines cause mice to increase their locomotor activity (amount of running). Any drug that blocks the effects of amphetamine on increased running in mice has a higher likelihood of working as an antipsychotic agent in schizophrenia. This is because amphetamine increases dopamine levels in mice, and drugs that block the effects of increased dopamine also tend to block hallucinations and delusions. Thus, the model has good predictive validity but poor face and construct validity. Several examples of behavioral models that have face, construct, or predictive validity for schizophrenia and its treatment are noted below.

Sensorimotor Gating

The term *sensorimotor gating* refers to a process in which a weak sensory stimulus (e.g., a faint sound) causes the inhibition of a subsequently elicited motor response (e.g., blink reflex) to a startling stimulus (e.g., loud sound). This process has been proposed as a model for the ability of a person to automatically filter out repetitive or persistent sensory information (Braff et al., 2001). For example, some patients report that they continue to hear background noises, like the hum of a fan or sound of traffic outside, rather than adapting to these sounds over time. Reduced sensorimotor gating has been observed in several psychiatric disorders, including but not limited to schizophrenia (Braff, Grillon, & Geyer, 1992). Although not specific, sensorimotor gating deficits may be particularly relevant to the study of schizophrenia. This linkage has been proposed because the ability of a drug to increase sensorimotor gating in rodent models predicts the clinical efficacy of medications used to treat positive symptoms such as hallucinations and delusions (Swerdlow, Braff, & Geyer, 2000). Some investigators have also suggested that symptoms experienced by patients with schizophrenia may result, in part, from the inability to filter sensory information (Geyer, Krebs-Thomson, Braff, & Swerdlow, 2001). There is also a high degree of conservation across species for biological processes involved in sensorimotor gating (Braff et al., 2001; Swerdlow et al., 2000). Therefore, mouse and rat models have been used to study sensorimotor gating using a task called prepulse inhibition of acoustic startle (PPI) in which the presentation of a nonstartling acoustic stimulus (prepulse, i.e., faint sound) inhibits the startle response elicited by a later startling stimulus (e.g., loud sound). The extent to which an animal inhibits the subsequent startle response is thought to reflect the animal's ability to filter or gate sensory information (Swerdlow et al., 2000). These studies suggest that several neurotransmitter systems, including dopamine, serotonin, and glutamate, regulate sensorimotor gating. This observation that several transmitter systems have similar effects suggests that there is convergence on a common biological mechanism or pathway to disrupt gating (Geyer et al., 2001).

Physiological Abnormalities

There are several behavioral and physiological markers of schizophrenia that are viewed as potential biological intermediaries linking the clinical diagnosis to its underlying neurobiological substrates. Auditory event-related potentials (ERPs) are among the most extensively studied intermediate markers of schizophrenia (Boutros et al., 1991; Clementz, Keil, & Kissler, 2004; Erwin, Mawhinney-Hee, Gur, & Gur, 1991; Freedman, Adler, Waldo, Pachtman, & Franks, 1983; Jin et al., 1997; Siegel, Waldo, Mizner, Adler, & Freedman, 1984; Umbricht et al., 1998). In these studies, an auditory stimulus evokes a series of electroencephalographic (EEG) brain responses corresponding to progression of brain activity throughout the auditory pathway. The auditory stimuli are presented many times (about 80 trials in most studies) while the continuous EEG is recorded. This EEG signal will include all brain activity occurring during the presentation of sounds, including the auditory responses as well as other brain activity. For example, all visual, olfactory, and tactile activity, as well as internally generated activity (thought) will be present. However, this nonauditory activity will be random with respect to the timing of the auditory stimulus. The EEG signal is then averaged across all trials to remove nonauditory activity, leaving only the activity that follows the stimulus in the same way in each trial. Any brain activity that is not exactly the same following each presentation of a sound will average to a value of zero and not contribute to the ERP. The pattern of activity that remains forms a series of peaks and troughs that are called components of the overall ERP. This is similar to naming the individual mountain peaks and valleys that make up a mountain range.

Early components (below 10 milliseconds) originate in the cochlea and auditory nuclei of the brainstem, while midlatency components including a positive deflection at approximately 50 ms in humans called the P50 (positive at 50 ms) reflect activation of the auditory thalamus and auditory cortex (Erwin et al., 1991; Picton & Hillyard, 1974; Picton, Hillyard, Krausz, & Galambos, 1974). Longer latency components including a negative deflection at approximately 100 ms in humans (N100) have been localized to come from the primary auditory cortex and cortical association areas (Gallinat et al., 2002). Abnormalities in the P50 and N100 components are postulated to reflect abnormal neuronal architecture and function. It is further postulated that abnormal modulation of auditory responses in patients may be informative about generalized neurological impairments in schizophrenia (Adler et al., 1998; Freedman et al., 1994).

Gating of ERPs

Many studies in schizophrenia have measured these ERP brain responses following a series of paired clicks. In these tasks, the amplitude of the EEG response to the first stimulus is normally larger than the response to the second. People with schizophrenia do not demonstrate this pattern of reduced response to the second click. Although this approach has been extensively applied to study the P50, it should be noted that multiple ERP components including the N100 also decrease in amplitude following the second stimulus (Boutros, Belger, Campbell, D'Souza, & Krystal, 1999; Boutros, Korzyukov, Jansen, Feingold, & Bell, 2004; Erwin et al., 1991; Erwin, Shtasel, & Gur, 1994; Rosburg, 2004). This is important because it suggests that patients have more widespread abnormalities through-out the brain, spanning systems from the brainstem to the thalamus and higher cortical regions. Most studies frame this abnormality as a failure to inhibit the second response in schizophrenia patients. As such, it is linked conceptually to a failure to adapt to persistent stim-uli in the environment, such as the noise from a fan or the sound of cars passing outside a window. There is, however, no association between the subjective report of not adapting to persistent sounds and failure to gate ERPs in individual patients.

Alternatively, several studies indicate that unmedicated schizo-phrenia patients actually have reduced amplitude of the P50 (rela-tive to normal controls) following the first stimulus in a paired click task with resulting loss in gating of the second (e.g., the sec-ond response is no smaller than the first) (Freedman et al., 1983; Jin et al., 1997). Thus, conceptually the abnormality becomes a failure to mount the normal response in the first place, rather than a failure to inhibit. Although this finding has been replicated in some studies of patients treated with antipsychotic medications, other studies indicate that antipsychotic treatment increases amplitude for both the first and second responses, maintaining the loss of gating (Clementz, Geyer, & Braff, 1998; Clementz et al., 2004; Freedman et al., 1983). This profile of equal amplitude of response to the first and second stimuli has been conceptualized as impaired gating (Adler et al., 1998).

Importantly, nicotine has been shown to restore gating among medicated schizophrenia patients. Some studies have attributed the effect of nicotine on gating to a reduction in the second re-sponse, while others indicate that nicotine acts primarily to in-crease the amplitude of the first (Figure 5.2) (Adler & Gattaz, 1993; Crawford, McClain-Furmanski, Castagnoli, & Castagnoli, 2002; Siegel et al., 2005). The observation that nicotine normalizes gating in patients has led to many pharmaceutical companies pur-suing nicotine-related compounds as possible therapies for schizo-phrenia. However, some data indicate that the beneficial effects of nicotine may be limited to medicated patients, suggesting it acts as

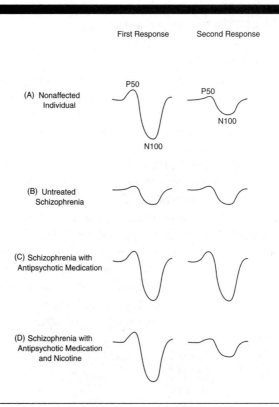

■ **Figure 5.2** Schematic representation of schizophrenia phenotypes for the P50 and N100.

(A) The normal pattern of P50 and N100 responses in nonaffected individuals. Note that the first response is large and the second is decreased. (B) In unmedicated schizophrenia, both the first and second responses are diminished for the P50 and N100. (C) Antipsychotic treatment results in increased amplitude of both the first and second responses for the P50 and N100 among schizophrenia patients, yielding the pattern of normal amplitude with impaired gating often described among medicated patients. (D) Nicotine reduces the amplitude of the second response among medicated schizophrenia patients.

an antidote for side effects rather than as a primary therapy for brain abnormalities in the illness (Siegel et al., 2005).

Physical Abnormalities

Several studies have demonstrated that physical abnormalities in schizophrenia may extend beyond brain anatomy. For example, minor physical anomalies are thought to include facial asymmetry, cleft palate, hair whorls, abnormal palmer crease, furrowed tongue, flat occiput, and primitive shape of ears (Gourion et al., 2004; Guy, Majorski, Wallace, & Guy, 1983; Sivkov & Akabaliev, 2003; Trixler, Tenyi, Csabi, & Szabo, 2001). One study found that 60% of schizophrenia patients and 38% of their siblings, but only 5% of control subjects, had a high rate of minor physical anomalies (i.e., six or more) (Ismail, Cantor-Graae, & McNeil, 1998). Several investigators have concluded that minor physical anomalies are an indirect index for early prenatal central nervous system maldevelopment, suggesting that schizophrenia results at least in part from neurodevelopmental damage (Green, Satz, Soper, & Kharabi, 1987; Hata et al., 2003). Furthermore, some studies have suggested that this relationship is most notable for males (Firestone & Peters, 1983; Green, Satz, Gaier, Ganzell, & Kharabi, 1989).

6 ▪ Current Medications

Historical Development of Antipsychotic Medication

The use of medicine for the treatment of schizophrenia dates back to 1952 with the serendipitous observation that chlorpromazine (Thorazine) yielded symptomatic improvement when given as a preanesthetic agent (Delay, Deniker, Harl, & Grasset, 1952; Delay, Deniker, & Harl, 1952; Shen, 1999). This was followed by the empiric discovery of other chemical entities with similar therapeutic effects. Approximately 10 years later, a seminal article by Seeman and colleagues documented that the clinically derived dose of all antipsychotic medications was highly correlated with the IC_{50} at striatal dopamine receptors (inhibitory concentration required for 50% reduction of some biological process) (Figure 6.1) (Seeman, Chau-Wong, Tedesco, & Wong, 1975; Seeman & Lee, 1975). A similarly important discovery resulted from complimentary evidence that agents that improved psychosis in schizophrenia resulted in increased dopamine metabolites in brain and cerebrospinal fluid (Carlsson & Lindqvist, 1963; Sedvall, 1980). These observations in total were the basis for the dopamine hypothesis of schizophrenia, which remains as valid today as it was then. The addition of in vivo imaging with positron emission tomography (PET) allowed further confirmation that therapeutic doses of antipsychotic agents resulted in approximately 70% to 80% dopamine D_2 receptor occupancy (Farde, Hall, Ehrin, & Sedvall, 1986; Farde et al., 1988). It must, however, be noted that all of these observations remain correlations, and dose finding for these medications is empirical rather than based on receptor affinity.

Clozapine

The next major advance in the treatment of psychosis resulted from the observation by John Kane and colleagues that clozapine (Clozaril) appeared to have superior efficacy as compared with

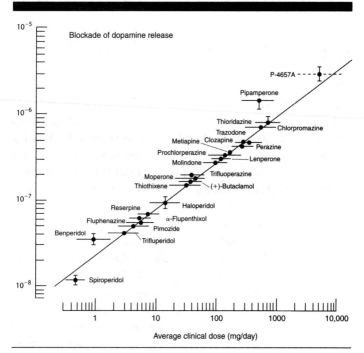

■ **Figure 6.1** The neuroleptic IC$_{50}$ values (the neuroleptic concentrations which inhibited the stimulated release of dopamine by 50%) correlate with the average clinical doses (in milligrams per day) for controlling schizophrenia.

The horizontal bars indicate the range of clinical doses. The vertical bars show the 20% variation in the IC$_{50}$ values. The correlation includes such diverse compounds as phenothiazines, butyrophenones, reserpine, pimozide, trazodone, clozapine, and (1)2 butaclamol. *Trans*-thiothixene (P-4657A) is of the order of one-hundredth the potency of its *cis*-isomer. Source: Seeman, M. Chau-Wong, J. Tedesco, K. Wong, Brain receptors for antipsychotic drugs and dopamine: direct binding assays. *Proc Natl Acad Sci USA.* (1975) 72 4376-80.

other agents among a population of treatment-resistant patients (Kane, Honigfeld, Singer, & Meltzer, 1988). One notable feature of this medication was that it also appeared to achieve significant improvement without the typical motor side effects seen with most other agents. This lack of motor side effects even at thera-peutic doses was unusual or "atypical" among existing medica-tions, leading to the term *atypical antipsychotic* for clozapine. Unfortunately, the term *atypical* medication took on broader meanings as it was applied to newer medications over time. For example, many theories have been put forward to suggest why clozapine displays efficacy without the same degree of dopamine blockade as other drugs. However, a close inspection of the data presented in the landmark Seeman and Lee article clearly show that clozapine sits squarely on the same correlation line as all other drugs for dopamine blockade and dose. Thus, the observation is more accurately stated that clozapine appears to have a lower degree of motor side effects despite the same level of dopamine blockade as other medications. Much attention was then placed on decomposing the receptor-binding profile for clozapine to dis-cover which receptor-binding properties might contribute to the relative lack of motor side effects. This led to initial hypotheses that the ratio of serotonin type 2 to dopamine type 2 receptor binding was a key feature of atypicality (Ereshefsky, Watanabe, & Tran-Johnson, 1989; Nordstrom, Farde, & Halldin, 1993; Nord-strom et al., 1995). However, this theory has failed to yield any medications that match clozapine in efficacy. Additionally, chlor-promazine (the first antipsychotic medication) actually meets this and many other definitions of "atypicality" since it has significant serotonin type 2 and dopamine type 2 binding at clinical doses (Trichard et al., 1998). A number of other theories have been put forward in an attempt to retain the idea that newer medications are categorically, mechanistically, or clinically distinguished from older ones. For example, one theory poses that "atypical" agents have less prolactin elevation than typical ones (Rauser, Savage, Meltzer, & Roth, 2001). However, risperidone, which is considered atypical, has among the highest prolactin elevation among all antipsychotic medications, and chlorpromazine, the original agent, has only moderate increases (Cheer & Wagstaff, 2004; Gruen et al., 1978; Kinon et al., 2003; Langer, Sachar, Gruen, & Halpern, 1977).

Similarly, several authors have hypothesized that "atypical" agents might improve cognition (Meltzer & McGurk, 1999). However, several studies have not found cognitive benefits for newer agents over older ones, and a recent large-scale comparison of newer agents versus the "typical" agent perphenazine (Trilafon) showed that the older, typical agent showed a slight but significant advantage over newer drugs for cognitive improvement (Keefe et al., 2005; Keefe, 2006; Siegel et al., 2006). Other definitions have similarly failed to distinguish any classlike properties among older (pre-risperidone, Risperdol) and newer (risperidone and newer) agents. Table 6.1 lists a summary of antipsychotic agents available in the United States, and Table 6.2 lists the receptor affinity for a subset of these medications (Seeman, Corbett, & Van Tol, 1997).

Chlorpromazine Equivalents

The term *chlorpromazine equivalents* indicates that doses of all antipsychotic medications can be normalized to a single scale based on potency. The scale is defined by how the clinically efficacious dose of each medication compares to the efficacious dose of all others. By convention, chlorpromazine is used as the standard because it was the first agent. For example, the system correctly notes that 100 mg of chlorpromazine is about as efficacious as 2 mg of haloperidol. Thus, haloperidol is 0.02 (2%) chlorpromazine equivalents (e.g., 500 mg of chlorpromazine will work about as well as 10 mg of haloperidol). All antipsychotic medications can be described in this manner using the maximum or average doses. There is a very high correlation between chlorpromazine equivalents and binding affinity at the dopamine D_2 receptor because antipsychotic efficacy is essentially a function of D_2 antagonism. However, it is a misconception to think that equivalents are based on, or determined by, binding affinities instead of clinical, empirical data. This system allows clinicians to estimate the dose of a new medication based on the dose a patient took of a previous one. For example, a patient switching from 4–6 mg of risperidone would need 15–20 mg of olanzapine or 8–12 mg of haloperidol for equivalent effect.

Table 6.1 List of Antipsychotic Medications

Medication	Category	Class	Metabolism	Prominent Side Effects	Prolactin Elevation	Daily Dose Range in mg	Frequency	Chlorpromazine Equivalents
Aripiprazole	Newer	Quinolinone	CYP450 2D6, 3A4	Insomnia, agitation, anxiety	Mild	10 to 15	Daily	0.02
Chlorpromazine	Older	Phenothiazine	CYP450 2D6	Sedation, hypotension, shuffling gait	Mild	200 to 800	Three times daily	1.00
Clozapine	Older	Dibenzodiazepine	CYP450 1A2, 2D6, 3A4	Sedation, tachycardia, sialorrhea	Low	300 to 600	Twice daily	0.75
Fluphenazine	Older	Phenothiazine	CYP450 2D5	Nausea, EPS	Moderate	0.5 to 10	Daily	0.01
Fluphenazine decanoate	Long-acting	Phenothiazine with 10 carbon ester linkage	CYP450 2D6	Nausea, EPS	Moderate	12.5 to 100 per month	Monthly	0.00

(continues)

Table 6.1 continued

MEDICATION	CATEGORY	CLASS	METABOLISM	PROMINENT SIDE EFFECTS	PROLACTIN ELEVATION	DAILY DOSE RANGE IN MG	FREQUENCY	CHLOR-PROMAZINE EQUIVALENTS
Haloperidol	Older	Butyrophenone	CYP450 2D6, 3A4, 2D6 inhibitor	EPS, akathisia	Moderate	1 to 15	Twice daily	0.02
Haloperidol decanoate	Long-acting	Butyrophenone with 10 carbon ester linkage	CYP450 2D6, 3A4	EPS, akathisia *	Moderate	50 to 100 monthly	Monthly	0.00
Loxapine	Older	Dibenzodiazepine	CYP450 unkown	EPS, sedation	Moderate	60 to 100	Twice daily	0.13
Molindone	Older	Dihydroindolene	CYP450 unkown	Sedation, EPS	Mild	50 to 200	Three times daily	0.25
Olanzapine	Newer	Thienobenzo-diazepine	CYP450 1A2, 2D6, 2C18	Weight gain, constipation	Mild	10 to 20	Daily	0.03
Olanzapine-rapidly dissolving	Newer	Thienobenzo-diazepine	CYP450 1A2, 2D6, 2C19	Weight gain, constipation	Mild	10 to 20	Daily	0.03

Perphenazine	Older	Phenothiazine	CYP450 2D6	EPS, sedation	Mild	8 to 64	Twice daily	0.08
Pimozide	Older	Diphenylbutyl-piperidine	CYP450 1A2, 3A4	Akathisia, EPS	Moderate	2 to 10	Twice daily	0.01
Quetiapine	Newer	Dibenzothiazepine	CYP450 3A4	Sedation	Mild	150 to 750	Twice to three daily	0.94
Risperidone	Newer	Benzisoxazole	CYP450 2D6	EPS, hypotension, hyperprolactinema	Severe	1 to 4	Daily	0.01
Risperidone microspheres	Long-acting	Risperidone in PLGA microsphperes	CYP450 2D6	EPS, hypotension, hyperprolactinema*	Severe	25 to 50 every 2 weeks	Bi-monthly	0.00
Thioridazine	Older	Phenothiazine	CYP450 2D6	Sedation, dry mouth, constipation	Mild	200 to 800	Twice to three daily	1.00
Thiothixene	Older	Thioxanthene	CYP450 unknown	Akathisia, EPS	Moderate	4 to 15	Twice daily	0.02
Trifluoperazine	Older	Phenothiazine	CYP450 unknown	Hypotension, EPS	Moderate	4 to 10	Twice daily	0.01
Ziprasidone	Newer	Benzothiazolyl-piperazine	CYP450 3A4	Sedation, headache	Mild	80 to 160	Twice daily	0.20

Table 6.2   Radioligand-Independent Dissociation Constants

	D_2	D_4	$5\text{-}HT_{2A}$	D_2: $5\text{-}HT_{2A}$ Ratio	D_2:D_4 Ratio
Chlor-promazine	0.66 ± 0.05	1.15 ± 0.04	3.5 ± 0.06	0.19	0.58
Clozapine	44 ± 8	1.6 ± 0.4	11 ± 3.5	4.00	28.00
Fluphenazine	0.32 ± 0.03	50 ± 10	80 ± 19	0.004	0.0064
Haloperidol	0.35 ± 0.05	0.84 ± 0.05	25 ± 8	0.014	0.42
Molindone	6 ± 3	2,400 ± 800	5,800 ± 1,300	0.001	0.0025
Olanzapine	3.7 ± 0.6	2 ± 0.4	5.8 ± 0.7	0.64	1.85
Risperidone	0.3 ± 0.1	0.25 ± 0.1	0.14 ± 0.1	2.14	1.2
Quetiapine	78 ± 28	3,000 ± 300	2,500 ± 600	0.03	0.026
Thioridazine	0.4 ± 0.12	1.5 ± 0.5	60 ± 15	0.007	0.27
Trifluperazine	0.96 ± 0.2	44 ± 6	135 ± 50	0.007	0.022

In nM ± SE

Although there were some efforts to move away from using the term *chlorpromazine equivalents* for newer agents, there is no rationale to distinguish older or newer medications on this scale. The movement to create a new system was driven by several factors including the misconception that equivalents reflected something other than the empirical dose used in practice, a misconception that D_2 antagonism was less relevant in newer agents than older ones, and an agenda to support the illusion that new agents acted through a fundamentally different mechanism than older ones. Since there is now overwhelming data that newer and older antipsychotic medications are indistinguishable in efficacy or mechanism, the system of equivalents is just as valid today as it was 30 years ago. Table 6.1 shows chlorpromazine equivalents for available antipsychotic medications.

■ Start Clozapine Early in the Course of Treatment—
Case Study 6.1

Source: Patient is a 17-year-old male referred for a second opinion and clinical consultation by his therapist.

History of present illness: The current episode began approximately 6 months prior to the interview when the patient was admitted to a psychiatric hospital after he ingested an excessive amount of Xanax. The patient denied that it was a suicide attempt, but records indicate that he admitted that it was a suicide attempt at the time. He experienced increasing depression following a breakup with a long-standing girlfriend leading to that incident. Records indicate that he had been in several car accidents around that time.

During his initial hospitalization in the spring, he reported auditory hallucinations as well as developing delusions about "Texas Marshals" wanting to harm him because they thought he was involved in a terror plot.

He received medication trials with a number of antipsychotic agents including quetiapine and risperidone with the addition of chlorpromazine for agitation. Although the risperidone and chlorpromazine had been effective at times, he remains psychotic presently on very high doses of risperidone. He had several subsequent hospitalizations with suicidal ideation that resulted in addition and modification of medications including trials of lithium, Depakote, Celexa, and Ativan.

He participated in partial hospital programs upon discharge from the hospital. At the end of last year, he was homeschooled with tutorial support to aid in his difficulties. Although now out of the hospital, he remains depressed and states that his depression is characterized by isolation and lack of happiness.

Developmental history: Patient was diagnosed with ADHD at 10 years of age, and was treated with Adderall at that time. He describes that he has never experienced remorse or guilt. Specifically, he noted he has beaten up other kids, hurting one badly and adding "he didn't really deserve it." He also stated that he lit a kitten on fire with friends and watched it burn to death while they trapped it in a trash can. He states neither of these events evoked any sense of remorse or guilt.

Medical history: As part of his workup for first-break psychosis, he had a CT and subsequent MRI, both of which were normal. He had an EEG that was consistent with the minor changes due to medication. He has not had formal neuropsychological testing, which I discussed with him and his parents and outlined below (assessment).

Social history: He had been actively engaged in school sports including football and social activities including romantic relationships until the current episode. His parents are divorced and both remain actively engaged in his life and now in his mental health care. Both parents participated in the evaluation and worked cooperatively on the patient's behalf during the interview. He has experimented with several drugs of abuse, most notably marijuana and alcohol.

Medication:

Chlorpromazine 300 mg hs
Risperidone 7 mg/day
Depakote 1500 mg/d
Prozac 50 mg/day
Cogentin as needed
Ativan as needed

Family history: There is a distant relative with unknown illness requiring psychiatric hospitalization. His grandmother also had post-partum depression.

Mental status exam:

Appearance: Normal grooming and hygiene, in age-appropriate clothing.
Behavior: He was engaged in the interview.
Speech: Normal rate and amount.

Mood: "Pretty even."

Affect: Restricted, but engaged, within normal range at times.

Thought Process: Linear and logical.

Thought Content: No suicidal or aggressive thoughts, no delusions presently. He does report having referential ideas regarding TV in past.

Perception: Continues to have auditory hallucinations, reporting some experiences during the interview. He notes they are mostly commentaries on him and others.

Insight: Poor; although he states there are no problems at school, his parents note that he has yet to bring home any homework and will sometimes just get up and leave class.

Judgment: Reasonable; he was willing to come for evaluation and has shared information with his parents.

Impulse control: No difficulties presently.

Cognition: Within normal range based on general interview; no formal testing done at this time.

Assessment: The patient is a 17-year-old male with 6 months of auditory hallucinations, delusion, and loss of function, consistent with a diagnosis of schizophrenia. He has had multiple depressive episodes, with no history of mania, suggesting that bipolar disorder cannot account for his psychosis. His psychosis is not consistent with psychotic depression since it persists during periods of normal mood. However, his depressive symptoms could be treated more aggressively to rule out that the degree of depression he experiences is contributing to his disability. He also has had comorbid drug use, most prominently marijuana. This is unlikely to account for the degree of disability and symptoms he has experienced.

Recommendations: Given the degree of disability and young age of onset, I would advocate changing his medication regimen to seek a simpler and more effective plan. There is no indication for Depakote, so that would be the agent I would recommend tapering first. Similarly, the combination of risperidone at 7 mg with an additional

300 mg of chlorpromazine is not ideal given the lack of symptom remission and high side effect burden/potential. Rather, my first option would be to move directly to clozapine. The rationale is that there are still no other agents that match it for efficacy, thereby giving the patient his best shot to find his highest level of function by getting there as soon as possible.

If he and his family accept that plan, I would suggest a very slow crossover with clozapine starting at 25 mg and increasing by 25 mg every 3 days until a dose of 500–800 mg/day as indicated by full resolution of his hallucinations. Because it would take 2 months to reach that dose, the risperidone and chlorpromazine can be divided into roughly 10 parts (1 mg of risperidone = 100 mg of chlorpromazine) and decrease by one unit for every 50 mg of clozapine that are added.

If, however, the family is not willing to use clozapine, there are two alternatives. First would be to use olanzapine in conjunction with a rigorous diet and exercise plan. The advantages include some potential benefits over risperidone in efficacy, a very high safety margin, and the ability to start at a full treatment dose and taper the risperidone/chlorpromazine over 1–2 weeks.

A second option would be to use one of the older midpotency agents such as perphenazine and cross-titrate over 1–2 weeks.

If he remains depressed on fluoxetine (Prozac), one might consider a more aggressive treatment with a tricyclic antidepressant (TCA) or monoamine oxidase inhibitor (MAOI). However, I would suggest leaving that aside for 6 months until after he is stable on either clozapine (best choice), olanzapine (my second choice), or perphenazine (or a similar midpotency agent).

My recommendation regarding neuropsychological testing is that it may identify specific areas of weakness and strength that would help guide areas for the patient to focus on. It may also provide a baseline cognitive measure on which his progression could be assessed. However, given the high expense, I also caution that it is unlikely to change diagnosis or treatment, so it is by no means something one needs to rush into.

▉ Optimizing Care with Clozapine vs.
Depot Formulations—Case Study 6.2

Source: The patient, his mother, and his father.

History of present illness: Patient is a 23-year-old, single white male with approximately a 5-year history of psychiatric illness. The patient notes he was fine in high school and had normal childhood and adolescent development. He joined the army after graduating from high school and completed approximately 7 weeks of the 8-week basic training period. At that point, he notes that he was brought to the hospital for reasons he cannot explain. He remained in the army's psychiatric ward for 5 weeks before being discharged. He has lived with his parents since that time.

Over the past 5 years, the patient has experienced a constant level of disability. He has, however, worked for periods of time as a certified nursing assistant. He lost his last job approximately 2 years ago and allowed his license to lapse by accident. He hopes to regain his certification and employment. He has experienced the TV sending him messages as well as auditory hallucinations, which he says his current medication (ziprasidone, 80 mg bid) reduces, but does not eliminate. He and his family note that he did much better while taking olanzapine. However, he experienced significant weight gain and had to discontinue that treatment. He also tried haloperidol, which he says he got as a shot in an ER and/or inpatient setting. His descriptions of the incident suggest an acute injection during a period of either agitation or disorganization. He states he did not like haloperidol. He has never received any depot formulations, nor has he tried oral treatment with risperidone or clozapine. He and his parents state that he has demonstrated a recurrent and consistent pattern of medication discontinuation when feeling better, always leading to a relapse and rehospitalization. Each of these episodes has required longer recovery than the previous episode, often with a lower level of function upon recovery than had been previously attained. They all concur that he is better now than he was during his last hospitalization but that he has not regained his prior level of function during the illness. He states that there have been times when his younger sister told him his sentences do not make sense. His parents also endorse periods of disorganized thought and speech when off medication.

Both parents add that he has had periods of fear and some social isolation but has remained empathetic and engaged with his family and close friends. He still socializes with high school friends on a regular basis and has had a girlfriend during the past 5 years.

Psychiatric and medical history: He states his mood fluctuates with his circumstances but does not describe periods consistent with either major depression or mania. He has no other comorbid psychiatric, neurological, or medical illnesses that could account for his psychotic symptoms or level of disability over the past 5 years. He is currently in treatment with a psychiatrist with whom he has good therapeutic rapport.

Family history: The patient's parents are divorced, but both remain intimately involved in his life. His father received a diagnosis of bipolar disorder over 20 years ago, which he does not have. He has gone 20 years untreated without a single episode, absolutely and unequivocally ruling out bipolar mood disorder.

Social history: Patient notes that he drank too much alcohol in high school at times. He does not drink at all now and does not use any illegal drugs. He lives with his father and is presently unemployed.

Mental status exam:

Appearance: Well groomed and appearing his stated age.
Behavior: Pleasant and interactive throughout the exam with good eye contact and rapport. He laughed appropriately at times, generally reflecting his sense that he had answered all of the questions countless times.
Speech: Normal in rate and rhythm.
Mood: "Pretty good."
Affect: Congruent with mood, full range affect.

Thought process: Mildly tangential.

Thought content: Remarkable only for past referential delusions, without suicidal or homicidal thoughts.

Perception: Notable for mild intermittent auditory hallucinations without well-formed content or pattern he can describe.

Insight: Limited, as evidenced by a repetitive pattern of medication discontinuation during periods of relative health coupled with his current preference not to take medication if possible.

Judgment: Fair currently, taking medication.

Assessment: Patient is a 25-year-old male with a 5-year history of hallucinations, delusions, and disorganization with concurrent disability in occupational function that cannot be ascribed to a mood or medical or neurological cause. Thus, his symptoms meet all criteria for a diagnosis of schizophrenia. His symptoms are partially controlled on Geodon, but not as well as they were on Zyprexa. Extreme weight gain from Zyprexa precluded its continuation. He has not achieved his former level of function during the illness. This may reflect a new, lower maximum level of function with each relapse, as has been described in the literature. Alternatively, it could reflect a growing body of evidence that newer medications are no more effective than several older ones. The patient has also displayed a consistent tendency to discontinue medication once he feels well, contributing to the pattern of intermittent relapses and rehospitalization. An ideal medication plan could incorporate an effective medication as well as addressing compliance issues.

Recommendations: The most effective antipsychotic treatment is clozapine. I discussed the relative merits and difficulties of engaging in clozapine with the patient and his parents. If he is willing to comply with the regulations and practices to use clozapine, it is the best choice to give him the best chance at achieving a higher quality of life. If he chooses to start clozapine, it should be initiated at 25 mg/day and increased by 25 mg every 2–3 days. Current medication should be reduced by about 20% per week after clozapine is above 100 mg such that the transition will take a total of 1 month, after which clozapine will continue to be increased to a dose of 400–600 mg. Clozapine levels should be checked after a dose of 400 mg to ensure it is not approaching toxic concentrations. If clozapine is not possible (and if compliance remains an issue), he would benefit from a depot formulation.

Haloperidol is the best for this approach, followed by fluphenazine, as these are monthly preparations that can be administered in 1 mL via a small-bore needle. He could start with either of these medications at 50 mg per month while reducing Geodon by 20% per week. If neither of those are acceptable to him, risperidone Consta is similar in efficacy to haloperidol, although it must be given every 2 weeks with supplies mailed directly to the physician (complicating the process). Any depot preparation is superior to any oral except clozapine; any of the three would be an improvement over his current oral medication as a long-term plan.

Although there have been effective medications for the positive symptoms of schizophrenia since the mid 1950s, there has been relatively little progress on effective treatments for the negative, cognitive, and functional domains. Recent large-scale multicenter studies and meta-analyses demonstrate that newer, formerly called *atypical*, medications have had little impact on improved efficacy, tolerability, or compliance with treatment. Additionally, nonadherence to existing medications significantly complicates treatment because the majority of patients do not take medication consistently. Future treatments will focus on both new mechanisms of action and improved delivery systems to target unmet needs in schizophrenia.

Goals of Therapy

The term *therapeutic goal* in schizophrenia must unfortunately be divided into *realistic goals* and *idealized or eventual goals*. Using current treatments, therapy for schizophrenia can realistically be expected to reduce positive symptoms such as hallucinations, delusions, and disorganization in about 70% of patients, most of the time (Dixon, Lehman, & Levine, 1995). This will usually be complicated by very low adherence rates in schizophrenia such that up to 70–90% of patients take their medications intermittently or erratically (Adams & Howe, 1993; Cramer, 1998; Valenstein, Copeland, Owen, Blow, & Visnic, 2001). Although estimates of nonadherence vary widely, a review of 39 studies found a mean nonadherence rate of 41.2%, and factors most consistently associated with nonadherence included poor insight, negative attitude or subjective response toward medication, previous nonadherence, substance abuse, shorter illness duration, inadequate discharge planning or aftercare environment, and poorer therapeutic alliance (Lacro, Dunn, Dolder, Leckband, & Jeste, 2002). This unfortunate pattern is so prevalent that adherence with medication is the major determinant of outcome for patients with schizophrenia today (Corriss et al., 1999). Additionally, every time patients relapse, they generally require higher doses of medication, and a longer duration to recover from each subsequent exacerbation. This, coupled with the observation that patients achieve a lower level of function with each relapse, may result from a combination of biological as well as social factors. Some theories propose that each relapse causes a toxic psychosis in which untreated schizophrenia includes a progressive brain deterioration such that the lack of medication allows progression of the brain abnormalities, leaving the patient with less brain reserve after each relapse. Additionally, each relapse has social consequences if patients manifest symptoms in their occupational, social, and or residential settings. For example, prior to onset, patients may be living independently, working, and have an ample network of friends. With the first episode they may loose their initial job, apartment, and some friends who witness their bizarre and frightening behaviors. After resolution of that episode, the patients may resume a similar level of functional potential, but will lose continuity of work history and the ability to use their former employer and landlord as references. Even if they are able to recover from the first episode, every time the patients cease medication and have a relapse, they will likely become cut off from another set of people. The more times these patients relapse, the more they burn bridges to society and become more isolated. This "social toxicity" compounds the biological toxicity making the patient both less functional and less integrated with possible support systems. If, alternatively, these patients continue to take their medication, they are far less likely to relapse and fall into this downward spiral. That said, "good" outcome for schizophrenia is still largely defined as an absence or minimal amount of positive symptoms with virtually no effect on negative symptoms or cognitive difficulties as discussed further below. A small percentage of patients, perhaps 10–15% or less, can achieve some level of significant functioning in family or vocational roles (Rosenheck et al., 2006). Optimal settings for these individuals include low-stress jobs that do not require a great deal of mental flexibility or multitasking, as these capabilities are usually quite impaired. Of note, there is also a perspective among the psychiatric community that medications cease to work over time as patients become resistant to their therapeutic effects despite good adherence. This latter observation suggests a biological progression of illness such that the previous level of treatment is no longer sufficient.

Pharmacologic Targets
Positive Symptom Domain

The most obvious characteristic of schizophrenia is the positive symptom cluster. As noted above, these symptoms are named for the presence of behaviors or sensations that should not be present. However, they could also be called "positive" because there is a positive response to medication. That is, most available medications dramatically reduce these symptoms in most patients most of the time. This is true for both the majority of older, "typical" agents and to a variable degree for newer "atypical" ones (Davis, Chen, & Glick, 2003; Geddes, Freemantle, Harrison, & Bebbington, 2000).

The treatment of positive symptoms appears to be related to antagonism of the dopamine D_2 type receptor. The D_2 receptor is a membrane bound G-protein (short for guanine nucleotide-binding proteins) that is linked to inhibition of adenylyl cyclase through its alpha subunit. When dopamine binds to the D_2 receptor, it leads to a cascade of events that decrease the activity of the enzyme adenylyl cyclase (AC). This in turn decreases formation of cyclic adenosine monophosphate (cAMP), which reduces the activity of another enzyme called protein kinase A (PKA, also known as cAMP-dependent protein kinase). The reduction of PKA activity reduces phosphorylation of many intracellular substrates including ion channels and DNA-binding proteins. Thus, in the presence of a D_2 receptor antagonist, this process is reduced, and there is an increase in intracellular cAMP and its downstream effects. There have been some limited efforts to recapitulate this effect using novel receptor-independent mechanisms including inhibition of the enzymes that degrade cAMP (Figure 6.2). These are limited thus far to basic science studies using animal models of schizophrenia (Maxwell, Kanes, Abel, & Siegel, 2004). However, these efforts have not yielded therapeutic interventions thus far.

Negative Symptom Domain

Although typical antipsychotic medications have long been known to reduce positive symptoms, they do not address the negative symptoms of schizophrenia. Early claims for new antipsychotic medications (those introduced since the early 1990s) included improved efficacy for negative symptoms (Remington, 2003). However, these claims have not been substantiated over time (Geddes et al., 2000; Lieberman et al., 2005). These newer drugs were formerly called "atypical" antipsychotic medications for a variety of reasons, including proposed efficacy for negative symptoms. However, the use of this definition of atypicality has diminished owing to a number of studies that found no difference between older and newer medications for negative symptoms. The term **primary negative symptom** refers to the reduction in normal emotion, motivation, and action that is due to the illness. This is distinguished from medication-induced or **secondary negative symptoms** that have been postulated to result from excessive doses

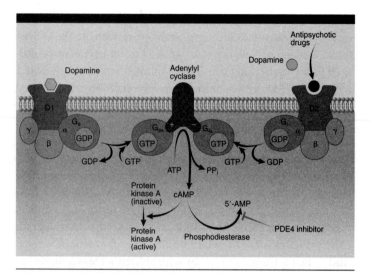

■ Figure 6.2   Schematic representation of the DA receptor-
                coupled adenylyl cyclase-cAMP pathway.

All current antipsychotic drugs are believed to work via antagonism at the
G-protein coupled D_2 dopamine receptor. Whereas D1/5 type DA receptors increase the activity of adenylyl cyclase (AC), D_2 dopamine receptors
decrease AC activity. AC is an enzyme that transforms adenosine triphos-
phate (ATP) to cyclic adenosine monophosphate (cAMP), which is a
ubiquitous intracellular second messenger. Furthermore, cAMP levels are
tightly controlled by phosphodiesterase (PDE) activity PDEs degrade the
cAMP molecule to 5′-AMP. Inhibition of PDE activity by PDE inhibitors
therefore increases cAMP levels. Thus, antagonism of the D_2 receptor with
antipsychotic medication and inhibition of PDE leads to increased cAMP
levels via different mechanisms. The ability to design new medications
requires an understanding of the biological systems that are abnormal in
schizophrenia. A clear understanding of specific biological abnormalities
would then help identify related targets for drug action. However, all
efforts to date have been based on the empiric observation that antagonism of the D_2 type dopamine receptor tends to work on positive symptoms. These agents (D_2 antagonists) have virtually no effect on negative
and cognitive symptoms.

of antipsychotic medication leading to either motor abnormalities (stiffness) or sedation. As doses have been lowered with changing standards of practice over the past 20 years, these difficulties have become less prominent. Because this change in practice has been coincident with the availability of new medications, it is difficult to distinguish the benefits of lower doses from reduced side effects due to improved medications.

Negative symptoms remain a major untreated dimension of schizophrenia. Additionally, residual negative symptoms result in significant functional impairment. The lack of efficacy for negative symptoms may reflect a loss of brain substrates (neuronal populations, connectivity, receptor systems) that are necessary for normal emotional and motivated behaviors by the time the diagnosis is made. In this scenario, negative symptoms reflect an immutable process that is resistant to any pharmaceutical intervention. A second possibility is that pharmaceutical development has simply not addressed the necessary neuronal substrates to treat negative symptoms. Specifically, the majority of animal models have been developed using dopamine agonists that have predictive validity only for positive symptoms (Geyer et al., 2001; Megens, Niemegeers, & Awouters, 1992; Schechter, 1980; Swerdlow, Braff, Taaid, & Geyer, 1994; Weiner, 2003). However, few models exist to screen compounds for negative symptom efficacy, with even fewer applied during pharmaceutical development (Corbett et al., 1993). Under this hypothesis, current preclinical screens may not only select for positive symptom efficacy but may actually exclude negative symptom efficacy by design. This would be true if dopamine D_2 receptor-mediated processes are not involved in negative symptom etiology. Therefore, the field needs to start applying validated animal models that predict negative symptom efficacy for new medications. This argument becomes circular as we have no agents that improve negative symptoms in humans and therefore no mechanism to validate predictive value for new animal models. Fortunately, the lack of preclinical screening tools to develop treatments for social and emotional deficits is starting to be addressed. For example, mouse models for abnormal social behaviors are now being developed to identify drug candidates and genes related to negative symptoms in schizophrenia and other illnesses (Figure 6.3) (Brodkin, 2005; Brodkin, Hagemann, Nemetski, & Silver, 2004).

Cognitive Symptom Domain

Similarly, current medications have little or no effect on other aspects of schizophrenia, such as cognitive deficits that contribute to the lifelong disability (Rosenheck et al., 2006; Siegel et al., 2006). As noted above, a great deal of effort has recently been placed on developing standardized batteries, such as the MATRICS, that can be applied across clinical trials to provide a clearer measure of cognitive efficacy. There are several traditional neurocognitive deficits in schizophrenia. Some are more heavily researched than others. Fundamental deficits in schizophrenia include impairments of visual processing, sustained attention, working memory, executive function, and general intelligence. Each of these domains is discussed below.

Visual Processing

The concept of visual processing pertains to the degree to which a person can identify and attend to features of a visual stimulus. For example, if you see a container of matches fall to the floor do you see it simply as a bundle of matches or can you process the full number at a glance? Most people can only process 6–7 items at a time, but if grouped into smaller units of 7 or less, they are able to make sense of a larger cluster. For example, it is easier to count a pile of marbles in multiples of 2s or 4s rather than processing a singular pile of 30. Healthy individuals are unable to attend to multiple items at one time, but when grouped into units ("chunking"), it is easier to process.

To gain a better understanding of how patients with schizophrenia create an internal representation of their surroundings, visual processing tests were designed. These tasks assess which relevant

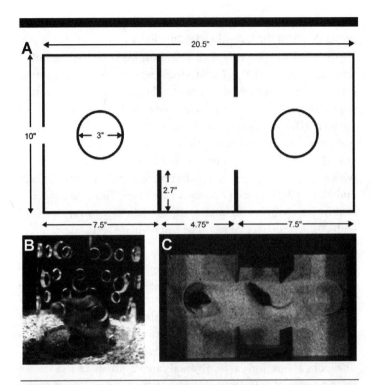

■ **Figure 6.3**   Behavioral testing apparatus scale.

(A) Dimensions of the behavioral testing apparatus. (B) Multiple small holes are evenly spaced over the entire surface of the cylinders in each end chamber. (C) The social approach—avoidance testing apparatus viewed from above. There is a clear Plexiglas cylinder in each of the two end chambers, and the center chamber is empty. Prior to the start of each test, one of the end chambers was arbitrarily designated the "social side" (the side into which the stimulus mouse would be introduced), and the other end chamber was designated the "nonsocial side."
Images provided by Dr. Ted. Brodkin.

details a patient with schizophrenia is able to pick up from a quick scan of the environment. One task designed to measure visual processing is called backward masking. In backward masking, a target image is flashed on a screen followed by another image intended to decode it (e.g., a *T* is flashed as a target and then masked by a group of 6 *X*s). When the second image, the mask (group of *X*s), is presented it tends to prevent the coding of the initial image (e.g., interference, in this case the *T*). Backward masking effects happen to everyone. However, individuals with schizophrenia and their first-degree relatives have a significantly increased deficit in backward masking. The mask appears to make it more difficult for someone with schizophrenia to identify the target image when it is later presented. This effect is thought to be determined by interactions within specific cell types that make up the so-called magnocellular and parvocellular visual pathways in the brain. Thus, masking procedures may help isolate specific cellular deficits pathways involved with this performance deficit in schizophrenia.

Sustained Attention

Sustained attention is the ability to direct and focus thoughts on specific stimuli while avoiding distractions. To complete any planned activity, sequenced action, or thought, one must use sustained attention. Significant problems occur when distractions arise and attention is broken. When testing sustained attention, one looks at how long an individual can pay attention to a task in the presence of interference, before their level of performance declines. Patients with schizophrenia show a deficit in sustained attention when compared to normal controls, but the exact nature of the deficit is not clear. One might assume that deficits in sustained attention would manifest as optimal performance at the beginning of a task followed by a reduction in performance over time. However, patients with schizophrenia do not differ from normal controls in vigilance. Rather, patients differ in overall sensitivity to distracters throughout the task. Thus, it is likely the basic mechanisms of attention rather than its endurance are impaired.

Selective Attention

Selective attention refers to one's ability to pay attention to stimuli of interest while ignoring other stimuli that is not of importance.

The classic example is the "cocktail party phenomenon" where two people can have a conversation despite a loud atmosphere and several other conversations and actions throughout the room. Patients with schizophrenia have a particularly difficult time with selective attention and are far more distractible than a normal control.

Memory

Memory can be broken down into verbal and nonverbal memory. When testing verbal memory, patients with schizophrenia display severe deficits in recall and to a lesser extent in recognition. For example, if a story is followed by a delay, patients are less likely to recall the initial story than nonaffected individuals. However, when presented with details of the story, they are able to distinguish items that may or may not have been present in the story easier than they are able to retell events.

Memory can be further broken down into implicit and explicit memory. Implicit memory is out of conscious control. An example of implicit memory is how you improve with practice when learning how to use a mouse on the computer. Studies suggest that implicit (procedural memory) is relatively intact in patients with schizophrenia when compared to explicit memory. Explicit memory is the type of recall for specific facts or events, as discussed above (e.g., recalling a list or a story), where deficits are severe in schizophrenia.

Working memory is a function of the prefrontal cortex and can be thought of as very short-term memory. Patients with schizophrenia have more difficulty than controls when required to retain information that is presented followed by a delay and are then asked to select the target stimulus among several possibilities. However, when no delay is presented, there is no significant difference in performance when compared to normal controls.

Executive Functions

Executive functions are daily life skills associated with the prefrontal cortex and involve neurocognitive activities such as planning, problems solving, mental flexibility, and the ability to attend to multiple tasks. Patients with schizophrenia have a particularly difficult time with executive functions in day-to-day life. The most common test used to measure executive function is the Wisconsin Card Sorting Test (WCST). Researchers at the University of Pennsylvania created a similar task that measures executive function as part of a computerized cognitive neuropsychological test battery (Web-CNP). In both the WCST and the CNP, the goal is to sort objects based on variables and rules that change throughout the test. The subjects are told that their response is "correct" or "incorrect" based on how they sort different objects into categories (e.g., shape, size, or color). After a number of consecutive "correct" choices, the rules change and a new sorting pattern is expected. Schizophrenia patients do poorly on these tasks more often than on other neurocognitive measures. An increased focus on executive function in recent years, with the aid of imaging studies, indicates that activation of the prefrontal cortex during working memory tasks is reduced in schizophrenia patients.

General Intelligence—IQ (Intelligence Quotient)

IQ scales do not assess some of the most crucial neurocognitive domains in schizophrenia. However, IQ tests are still widely used because of their large databases of information gathered in the past—particularly in school and hospital settings. Schizophrenia patients tend to score lower than would generally be expected of the individuals based on their family and environmental structure. Patients tend to have higher verbal IQ, in comparison to performance IQ scores. Reduction in IQ is also found among prodromal adolescents, albeit increasing in severity at the onset of illness and then stabilizing. Reduced IQ among prodromal individuals may be interpreted in several ways. An individual with a high IQ may have increased internal resources to cope with stressors on a different level than someone with a lower IQ. Thus, IQ may be an indicator of the individual's ability to cope with stressful life events and modulate the likelihood of surpassing the threshold for disease to manifest. Alternatively, lower IQ could simply be a biomarker for the genetic predisposition to develop schizophrenia.

Generalized Neurocognitive Deficits—Explanations

Overall, schizophrenia patients have deficits in multiple domains of cognitive function. However, these patients do not perform equally poorly on all measures or domains of cognitive function. Specifically, patients have relatively greater deficits in memory, especially while being distracted. Additionally, schizophrenia patients have more difficulty with recall than recognition, suggesting that retrieval rather than encoding of information is the main deficit. The field continues to search for mechanisms of these deficits that could help identify a strategy to aid in better understanding, diagnosis, treatment, and early intervention for cognitive abnormalities.

Emotional and Social Cognition

Recently, more attention has been directed at nontraditional cognitive domains including social and emotional intelligence. These concepts refer to the innate ability to comprehend, process, and respond to emotional and social cues. Much of the communication among people is conveyed using nonverbal cues and signals including facial expressions, body language, and intonation. Clinicians have long recognized that patients with schizophrenia often lack these basic social skills. Additionally, these patients appear to lack the basic understanding and interpretation of such nonexplicit or nonsemantic forms of communication. Several research studies have attempted to quantify such deficits using scales in which patients rate the emotional expression on a photograph of a facial expression. These studies suggest that patients have difficulties both identifying the appropriate expression and ascribing intensity to these expressions. Thus, patients' relative inability to interact in social situations may result from their basic lack of understanding of the means of communication. Several programs are currently underway to teach social cognition to patients in an effort to explicitly help them recognize features that come intuitively to most people. In doing so, the hope is that patients with schizophrenia can learn to recognize specific emotions and nonverbal cues in others. Similarly, efforts are underway to teach patients how to make the appropriate facial and postural expressions in the service of "acting normal" to foster better interpersonal skills and function.

Therapeutic Approach

There is little consensus regarding the best approach to choosing an antipsychotic medication for a specific patient. Some experts have advocated the use of newer medications based on early reports that these agents had either greater therapeutic benefit or reduced side effects. However, the benefit of these agents in a subset of industry-sponsored clinical trials has been disputed by some clinicians. One caveat to this controversy is the widely held belief that clozapine remains unparalleled in efficacy. A limitation in the use of clozapine is that it is also unparalleled in side effect burden and logistic difficulty for both the patient and physician. Side effects of clozapine include a high degree of sedation, excessive salivation while sleeping, constipation, urinary retention, and rapid heart rate due to blockade of the cholinergic input to the heart. Although these side effects are the most common and disabling aspect of clozapine, there is also a very rare potential complication of treatment that leads to the logistic difficulties in taking it. Specifically, clozapine requires a weekly blood test to assess for a rare complication called agranulocytosis, in which patients can have suppression of their white blood cells. Each blood test result must be reviewed by a physician, documented on registry forms, and sent to the pharmacy so they may dispense a 1-week supply. After 6 months without an incident of agranulocytosis, patients may change to monthly blood tests in order to receive a 30-day supply. Titration of clozapine is extremely slow, because patients can develop delirium if one increases too quickly. The initial dose is 25 mg and can be increased by 25 mg every 3 days. A minimal therapeutic dose of clozapine is approximately 400–800 mg. Therefore, it takes 8–12 weeks to arrive at the therapeutic dose, requiring very slow cross-titration and discontinuation of whichever medication the patient was previously taking. These factors, side effects and logistics together, continue to cause the gross underutilization of clozapine among patients that could benefit from its superior efficacy. Several large meta-analyses and clinical trials have now shown that clozapine remains superior to all other agents, with small advantages for olanzapine (Zyprexa) and risperidone (Risperdol) over older medications for some domains and small advantages for newer medication over all newer ones on other domains (Figure 6.4) (Davis et al., 2003; Geddes et al., 2000; Keefe, 2006; Lieberman et al., 2005).

Therefore, the main factor in choosing a medication is generally based on matching of side effect liability with both patient and physician preferences and risk tolerance. For example, a number of medications that work well for positive symptoms such as haloperidol and risperidone have a relatively high risk of causing motor side effects such as stiffness and tremor as well as a feeling of restlessness called akathisia. These risks can be dramatically reduced by the use of low doses (e.g., 3–4 mg/day of risperidone or 4–8 mg/day of haloperidol). Additionally, there are countermeasures, including the use of anticholinergic medications such as benztropine that block the manifestation but not root causes of motor side effects. There are two distinct approaches to the use of anticholinergic medication based on the patient's and physician's risk tolerance. One approach favors starting the antipsychotic alone, without coadministration of anticholinergic medication to minimize unnecessary medication exposure. In this strategy, one can warn the patient that he or she may experience stiffness or tremor, but that you will be able to give an "antidote" if this should occur. The alternate approach is to start anticholinergic medication immediately as prophylaxis to minimize the chances that the patient will have an unpleasant experience. The latter approach

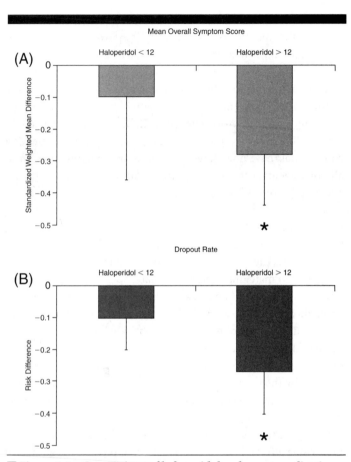

■ **Figure 6.4   Comparison of haloperidol and newer medications.**

(A) Overall symptom score by dose of comparator drug in trials of patients with schizophrenia or related disorders (standardized weighted mean difference and 95% confidence intervals). Note, that there is no difference between agents in studies when the dose of haloperidol was properly set at less than 12 mg. However, newer agents were superior to haloperidol when haloperidol's dose was set above the recommended level for the study. (B) Drop out rates by dose of comparator drug in trials of patients with schizophrenia or related disorders (risk difference and 95% confidence intervals). As noted for symptoms scores, haloperidol was equal to newer agents when appropriately dosed, but not when overdosed. Adapted from Geddes et. al., *BMJ*, 2000.

leads to risk of the anticholinergic side effects of dry mouth, constipation, and possibly cognitive impairment, which have sometimes been then inappropriately attributed to the antipsychotic medication. This effort to minimize antipsychotic side effects may also lead some clinicians to apply the strategy inappropriately by using benztropine in concert with medications for which it is not indicted. For example, olanzapine has high affinity as an antagonist at muscarinic acetylcholine receptors, likely accounting for its lower motor side effect risk. Therefore, additional anticholinergic medication is unlikely to be indicated. Conversely, olanzapine's liability is that it causes patients to lose their sense of satiety when eating, yielding increased appetite and weight gain of 20 pounds or more. Pharmacological countermeasures for this unfortunate and potentially deleterious side effect include off-label use of appetite suppressants such as topirimate (Topamax). However topirimate has its own serious side effects including profound memory disturbances. Therefore the use of topirimate to counter the appetitive problems with olanzapine is not often recommended. This leaves only behavioral countermeasures such as diet and exercise. Although these measures are completely effective if used, patients with schizophrenia are no more likely to adhere to proper eating and physical activity programs than the general public, which is quite poor at both. Despite the concerns above, physicians still tend to use medications of habit, coupled with loose guidelines of avoiding olanzapine in obese patients and risperidone or other high-potency agents in patients with a history of, or existing, severe motor problems.

There have been few efforts to create an evidence-based algorithm for initiation and maintenance of medication for schizophrenia. The only clear decision is that all patients need some form of medication all of the time. There has been one major initiative to provide guidelines for treatment. Although the **Texas Algorithm** was created prior to widespread realization that newer agents held little if any advantage over older ones, it does provide a strategy for treatment (Miller et al., 2004). One possible concern with this algorithm is that it does not distinguish among more and less efficacious medications. Rather, this algorithm gives preference to newer medications that many practitioners would argue are actually less effective and have higher side effect liability than many older ones (Figure 6.5).

To address this potential limitation in the Texas Algorithm, one of the authors (Siegel) has proposed an alternative algorithm based on clinical experience and literature (Figure 6.6). This algorithm is based on the following basic principles and hypotheses:

1. Clozapine is the most efficacious agent available, albeit one with many side effects that is difficult for patients to take.
2. There is a slight advantage for either risperidone or olanzapine over haloperidol and other older agents in large meta-analyses studies.
3. Other new antipsychotic medications do not offer substantial benefit and may actually be worse than older agents in some respects including both efficacy and side effects.
4. Nonadherence to medication is the major cause of all treatment failures; injectable long-acting agents should be used early in the therapeutic progression.

Of note, aripiprazole (Abilify) is relatively new at the time of this book's publication, so its role in treatment remains unclear. Thus far, one observation that seems clear is that more is not necessarily better beyond the recommended doses for any agent. This is perhaps most pertinent for the partial dopamine agonist aripiprazole, which takes on characteristics of a full dopamine agonist above about 15 mg in a 60–70 kg person. Thus, many people find that higher doses of aripiprazole are actually less effective than lower doses. Also, while many clinicians find quetiapine and ziprasidone less aggressive treatments than other agents, quetiapine is among the most prescribed medications in psychiatry, largely outside of schizophrenia due to its relative paucity of side effects and calming nature. Similarly, several reports have suggested ziprasidone may be useful in other disorders, such as bipolar disorder with psychosis.

Choice of antipsychotic (AP) should be guided by considering the clinical characteristics of the patient and the efficacy and side effect profiles of the medication.

Any stage(s) can be skipped depending on clinical picture or history of antipsychotic failure, and returning to an earlier stage may be justified by history of past response.

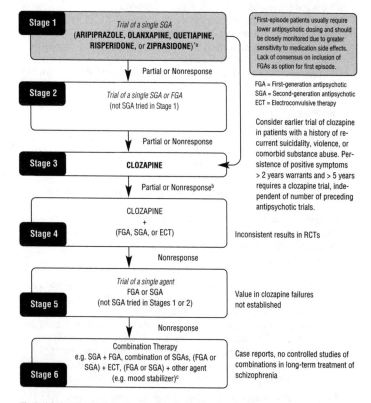

Stage 1
Trial of a single SGA
(ARIPIPRAZOLE, OLANXAPINE, QUETIAPINE, RISPERIDONE, or ZIPRASIDONE)[*][a]

*First-episode patients usually require lower antipsychotic dosing and should be closely monitored due to greater sensitivity to medication side effects. Lack of consensus on inclusion of FGAs as option for first episode.

↓ Partial or Nonresponse

Stage 2
Trial of a single SGA or FGA (not SGA tried in Stage 1)

FGA = First-generation antipsychotic
SGA = Second-generation antipsychotic
ECT = Electroconvulsive therapy

↓ Partial or Nonresponse

Stage 3
CLOZAPINE

Consider earlier trial of clozapine in patients with a history of recurrent suicidality, violence, or comorbid substance abuse. Persistence of positive symptoms > 2 years warrants and > 5 years requires a clozapine trial, independent of number of preceding antipsychotic trials.

↓ Partial or Nonresponse[b]

Stage 4
CLOZAPINE
+
(FGA, SGA, or ECT)

Inconsistent results in RCTs

↓ Nonresponse

Stage 5
Trial of a single agent FGA or SGA (not SGA tried in Stages 1 or 2)

Value in clozapine failures not established

↓ Nonresponse

Stage 6
Combination Therapy
e.g. SGA + FGA, combination of SGAs, (FGA or SGA) + ECT, (FGA or SGA) + other agent (e.g. mood stabilizer)[c]

Case reports, no controlled studies of combinations in long-term treatment of schizophrenia

[a]If patient is inadequately adherent at any stage, the clinician should assess and consider a long-acting antipsychotic preparation, such as resperidone microspheres, haloperidol decanoate, or fluphenazine decanoate.
[b]A treatment refractory evaluation should be performed to reexamine diagnosis, substance abuse, medication adherence, and psychosocial stressors. Cognitive Behavioral Therapy (CBT) or Psychosocial augmentation should be considered.
[c]Whenever a second medication is added to an antipsychotic (other than clozapine) for the purpose of improving **psychotic** symptoms, the patients is considered to be in Stage 6.

■ **Figure 6.5** **Algorithm for the treatment of schizophrenia.**

Texas algorithm has been among the first major efforts to operationalize treatment recommendations based on expert consensus. The major limitation to this approach is that it favors newer agents. The preponderance of data now clearly demonstrates that there is no benefit for efficacy, side effects, tolerability of functional/cognitive outcome from new agents. Therefore, the tendency to start with more expensive, newer medications is unjustified by evidence based practice principles.
TIMA SCZ, Algo Rev Jan 1996.

- **Background**: These guidelines are based on the following practices:
  - If the patient is well, do not change medications.
  - If the patient is experiencing symptom exacerbation or has a history of nonresponse to treatment, proceed to stage 1.
  - While changing medication, patients should be seen by a physician every 2 weeks for at least 6 weeks.
  - All patients that have not had a workup for psychosis should have the following tests. A subset of these tests (*) are instrumental in determining antipsychotic choice.
    - *Physical exam
      - □ Neurological exam for EPS
      - □ Signs of systemic illnesses with psychiatric manifestations
    - *Chemistry Panel 7
    - CBC with diff, LFTs, TSH, RPR, ANA
    - Toxicology screen
    - MRI to rule out intracranial inflammation, masses, and lesions

- **New onset: (patient not on any medication)**
  - Stage 1—*Olanzapine* if BMI under 25 and/or fasting glucose under 110
    - Begin at 10 mg/day and increase by 5 mg/week as indicated (based on 75 kg person, max 0.3 mg/kg/day)
    - Titrate to treatment dose within 2–3 weeks
    - Continue full dose for an additional 4 weeks to determine response
      - □ If responds to olanzapine, then continue at full treatment dose for 4 months before evaluating for lower dose.
      - □ If intolerable weight gain with good treatment response, consider intensive diet and exercise plan and/or appetite suppressant.
      - □ If poor treatment response to olanzapine, then cross-titrate to risperidone by decreasing olanzapine by 10 mg/wk while bringing risperidone to full treatment dose over 2 weeks as indicated below.

  - Stage 2—*Risperidone* if BMI over 25 and/or fasting glucose over 110
    - Begin at 2 mg/day and increase by 1 mg/week as indicated (based on 75 kg person, max 0.1 mg/kg/day)
    - Titrate to treatment dose within 2–3 weeks
    - Continue full dose for an additional 4 weeks to determine response
      - □ If responds to risperidone, then continue at full treatment dose for 4 months before evaluating for lower dose.
      - □ If unacceptable EPS with good treatment response, add benztropine 1 mg per day and titrate to 1 mg twice a day as needed.

■ **Figure 6.6** Algorithm for antipsychotic treatment.

☐ If poor treatment response to risperidone, then cross-titrate to haloperidol by decreasing risperidone by 3 mg/wk while initiating haloperidol as listed below.

◦ Stage 3—*Haloperidol*
  ▪ Begin haloperidol at 6 mg/day and increase by 2 mg per week as indicated (based on 75 kg person, max 0.2 mg/kg/day.)
  ▪ Titrate haloperidol to treatment dose within 2–3 weeks.
  ▪ Continue full dose for an additional 4 weeks to determine response.
    ☐ If responds to haloperidol, then continue at full treatment dose for 4 months before evaluating for lower dose.
    ☐ If poor treatment response to due to poor compliance then advance to Stage 4.
    ☐ If nonresponse to risperidone and/or haloperidol with severe motor side effects, then advance to Stage 5—Clozapine.

◦ Stage 4—*Depot injection* (treatment failure due to suspected or known noncompliance)
  ▪ Risperidone Consta—initiate at 25 mg IM every 2 wks while decreasing oral haloperidol by 6 mg/day/week.
    ☐ Increase dose to 50 mg every 2 weeks if partial response after 4 weeks.
    ☐ Evaluate response to Risperidone Consta after 8 weeks (three injections to reach steady state).
    ☐ If nonresponse to risperidone Consta and there is no severe adverse event on oral haloperidol, then cross-titrate to either fluphenazine or haloperidol decanoate by stopping risperidone Consta injections and initiating haloperidol decanoate as indicated below.
    ☐ Begin at 50 mg IM once per month and increase by 25 mg/month for 2 more months as indicated to max of 100 mg based on 75 kg person (1.33 mg/kg/mo).
    ☐ Evaluate long-acting depot after 3 months.
      ◦ If nonresponse to either fluphenazine or haloperidol decanoate, then advance to Clozapine.

◦ Stage 5—*Clozapine*
  ▪ Begin at 25 mg/day and titrate to treatment dose within 4–6 weeks by increasing dose by 25–50 mg every 2–3 days (100 mg/week) as tolerated, max dose 8 mg/kg/day divided bid.
  ▪ Check serum clozapine level after 4 weeks and again at final dose.
  ▪ Continue treatment dose for an additional 4 weeks to determine response.
  ▪ If nonresponse to clozapine, augment with haloperidol decanoate.

▪ **Figure 6.6** **Continued.**

- **Previously Treated Patients:**
  - ☐ History of **noncompliance**—go directly to **Stage 4** above
  - ☐ Follow to Stage 5 if both haloperidol and risperidone depot fail.
  - ○ If no history of noncompliance:
    - ■ Begin with Stage 1 above unless documented treatment failure on 20 mg/day olanzapine for 4 weeks.
      - ☐ Evaluate BMI and fasting glucose.
      - ☐ If BMI over 25 or fasting glucose over 110, proceed to Stage 2.
      - ☐ If only contraindication to olanzapine is history of weight gain (not frank obesity), consider initiating diet and exercise plan with appetite suppressant coadministration.
      - ☐ If olanzapine fails (either previously or following stage 1), then initiate Stage 2.
    - ■ Risperidone
      - ☐ Evaluate for presence or history of severe EPS, dystonia or neuroleptic malignant syndrome (NMS) (see page 162).
      - ☐ If motor problems or dystonia present, initiate coadministration of benztropine. If history of NMS, consider moving directly to clozapine.
      - ☐ If risperidone fails, proceed to Stage 3.
    - ■ Haloperidol
      - ☐ Evaluate for presence or history of severe EPS, dystonia, or NMS.
      - ☐ If motor problems or dystonia present, initiate coadministration of benztropine.
      - ☐ If haloperidol fails, proceed to Stage 4; if there is a history of NMS, proceed to Stage 5.
    - ■ Depot medication
      - ☐ If history of NMS or motor problems that could not be controlled with benztropine, proceed to Stage 5.
      - ☐ If depot trials of risperidone and haloperidol fail, proceed to Stage 5.
    - ■ Clozapine—follow instructions above.

■ **Figure 6.6   Continued.**

Treatment Response

Typical Pattern of Relapse and Recovery—CASE STUDY 6.3

Source: Patient, his mother, father, and sister.

History of present illness: Patient described the onset of difficulties 8 years ago, at which time he was admitted to a hospital. He and his family describe an initially difficult period at the hospital during which time he was given haloperidol, lithium, thioridizone (Mellaril), and Cogentin, after which they state he did exceedingly well while taking Clozaril 250 mg per day until December of last year. After 7 years of stability on Clozaril, the patient made a transition to quetiapine over a 2-week period with cross-titration in an effort to achieve similar efficacy without biweekly blood tests and to decrease risk of adverse side effects. However, according to all sources, he did not tolerate this transition and experienced a relapse within 4 weeks with reemergence of auditory hallucinations. Patient noted to have mood swings and had become frightened. Quetiapine was increased to a final dose of 400 mg daily, and Clozaril was reinstated at an initial dose of 200 mg and was titrated to 300 mg daily over the next few days. Clozaril increased to 400 mg and subsequently to 500 mg qd within 6 months of reinstatement. His current dose is 600 mg qd. Additionally, lithium (450 mg qd) as well as lorazepam (0.5 mg bid) were added. Despite alterations in dosing schedule of medications, he continued to experience auditory hallucinations of an unpleasant nature commanding him to turn off a mail-processing machine at work. He also developed mood swings and persecutory ideas resulting in medical leave beginning 1 week prior to our visit. The patient and his family present with an inquiry regarding the treatment strategies available.

Medical history: Hypothyroidism treated with Synthroid 0.075 mg/d

Social history: The patient describes normal childhood development, completed high school, after which he worked at Sears for several years followed by his current job where he is employed at the postal service. He lives alone in a condominium near his parents and has recently stayed with them during a difficult time. He has no drug or alcohol use problems.

Mental status exam:

Behavior: Patient was pleasant and cooperative without behavioral disturbances.

Affect: Bright.

Speech: Normal volume and rate.

Mood: "Better, but still sad."

Thought process: Tangential at times.

Thought content: Remarkable for ideas of having brought a coworker back from the dead; no thoughts of self-harm or harm to others. He states that in the distant past he told a coworker that he would come in the back door at work with an AK-47 but adds that it was a joke and that there were no repercussions of the statement.

Perception: No abnormalities present during interview.

Insight: Good.

Judgment: Good: "I'll take some time to get well before going back to work."

Mini Mental Status Exam: Revealed concrete interpretation of idioms; otherwise, no cognitive deficits apparent for recall, recognition, or attention.

Assessment: Patient is a 39-year-old male who had his first psychotic break 8 years ago at the age of 31. He had a good recovery and was initially able to resume a normal level of function. He was maintained on Clozaril 250 mg daily for the following 7 years. Unfortunately, he made an effort to switch medications in an effort to have less side effects and to not have routine blood tests. Although the patient had done quite well on a low dose of Clozaril, the attempt resulted in relapse with subsequent difficulty regaining stability.

Despite the apparent lack of efficacy of Clozaril prior to this evaluation, both the patient and his family indicate that he has improved during the days prior to our meeting. Subsequent conversations with the patient as well as his parents indicate continued improvement.

Recommendation: It is common that people need longer periods to recover after a second exacerbation than they had after an initial episode. As such, it is likely that the patient will continue to improve on his current regimen of medications. Additionally, full response may require as long as 1 year in some cases after a relapse.

In the event that he continues to improve, I recommend discontinuation of Ativan initially, followed by removal of lithium. I then recommend maintenance on Clozaril at stabilization dose (currently 600 mg/day) for a period of 4–6 months before tapering. If side effects become problematic, I recommend tapering Clozaril slowly over several weeks as tolerated.

In the event that Clozaril does not achieve remission, a trial of olanzapine remains an option with dosing starting at 10 mg per day and increasing up to 20 mg per day for a period of 6 weeks to assess an adequate trial.

Side Effects: Medical Comorbidities Caused by Medication

Side effects to antipsychotic medication include neurologic, endocrine, metabolic, and cardiac abnormalities. No medication is free from some combination of these effects, nor does any medication have a high side effect burden that rivals untreated illness for morbidity or mortality.

Neurological side effects include motor side effects such as stiffness, tremor, and akathisia. Stiffness usually results from excessive doses of high-potency agents such as risperidone or haloperidol. However, many medications can cause this effect in sufficiently high doses. Tremor, typically of a cog-wheel type, also results from higher potency agents, and is likely due to blockade of dopamine receptors in the striatum. *Akathisia* is the term for an inner sense of restlessness, generally thought to be the most unpleasant of all side effects, and most commonly sited by patients as a reason to discontinue a medication. Although less common, seizures represent a more severe form of neurological side effects for any antipsychotic medication. Although all such medicines lower seizure threshold, clozapine is by far the most common agent to cause this effect. Because of this possibility, clozapine levels should be monitored during dose titration and annually thereafter to ensure that serum levels remain below 1000 ng/mL since seizures become much more common above this level. Another severe, potential neurological complication of antipsychotic medication is called neuroleptic malignant syndrome (NMS). This constellation of reactions includes high fever, stiffness, elevated blood pressure, and other signs of autonomic instability. If one suspects NMS, the patient should go to an emergency room immediately as NML has a very high mortality, with estimates as high as 10% even with rapid admission to a medical intensive care unit.

Endocrine side effects include elevations in prolactin due to disinhibition of the pituitary. Men can develop gynecomastia, and women will lactate. Serum levels can exceed 100 ng/mL, with normal values of approximately 4 ng/mL for a man, and up to 30 ng/mL for a nonpregnant woman. Risperidone is among the most frequent medications to cause this particular effect, but it can occur with any higher-potency agent.

Metabolic effects include weight gain and possibly glucose resistance. Some research indicates that medications such as olanzapine and clozapine can cause a weight-independent increase in the incidence of type II diabetes. However, good diet and exercise is very effective in controlling both weight gain and serum glucose levels. Alternatively, the propensity to gain weight on olanzapine in particular seems more likely to be mediated by a central effect on appetite since virtually all patients that take it report dramatic increases in appetite and food intake. In such cases, there is obviously an increase in body mass index with resulting type II diabetes secondary to increased adipose tissue. Thus, the challenge is for patients and their families to resist increasing caloric intake just because the person is hungry. If this can be accomplished, the risk of weight gain and diabetes is averted entirely.

Cardiac complications include an increase in QTc due to calcium channel blockade (QT prolongation) and anticholinergic effects (rate acceleration). Virtually all antipsychotic medications cause QT prolongation. However, rate acceleration can be averted through the use of high-potency agents such as haloperidol or risperidone. Thus, these two agents are the drugs of choice for any patient with cardiac comorbidity.

Metabolism—Internist/Endocrinologist

◼ **Olanzapine-Induced Weight Gain**—Case Study 6.4

Source: Patient, his father, and records.

History of present illness: Patient is a 29-year-old male who first experienced auditory hallucinations while working as a runner in the stock market after graduating from college. Now treated effectively with olanzapine 15 mg po qhs as well as Wellbutrin (he doesn't know dose) for over 1 year. However, he has gained approximately 100 lb. He has been without symptoms for 1 year, until several days prior to this evaluation when he reported transient "paranoid feelings." In the past the patient believed that the CIA or FBI was involved in the voices, but now says he "never bought into that." He states that he does not socialize much and "doesn't like to work." He has mild difficulty concentrating on tasks such as keeping notes.

Medical history: No history of any medical illnesses.

Medications: Olanzapine 15 mg po qhs and Wellbutrin (doesn't remember the dose).

Psychiatric history: The patient began seeing a new psychiatrist near his home and recently enrolled in a vocational training program to acquire skills. He was an inpatient several years ago, at which time he received the diagnosis of schizoaffective disorder—full records from this admission were available. Additionally, he was treated as an outpatient, again with diagnosis of schizoaffective disorder.

Mental status exam:

Behavior: He is pleasant and personable with no behavioral abnormalities.

Speech: Normal.

Mood: "Good."

Affect: Full range.

Thought process: Logical.

Thought content: Without suicidal or homicidal thought. He retains strong religious beliefs regarding the Virgin Mary and God, but does not endorse any ideas outside the cultural norm for his religious group.

Perception: Denies abnormalities.

Insight and judgment: Good.

Assessment: Patient is a 29-year-old, single white male living with his parents. His history is remarkable for delusions and hallucinations, consistent with schizophrenia. Records indicate a prominent affective component during most extreme periods of illness, including both manic and depressive periods. Therefore, we concur with the previous diagnosis of schizoaffective disorde—type 1. Similarly we concur with current medications. Although there is a considerable risk of extreme weight gain with olanzapine, as this patient has experienced, its efficacy in him may warrant continuation.

Recommendations:

1. Continue olanzapine with addition of a formalized weight-reduction program including exercise and diet. Specifically, join a monitored program to aid with foods and eating patterns.
2. Continue vocational training to reintegrate into work, while avoiding high-stress environments like his previous job and capitalizing on his personality.
3. Obtain medical examination from internist regarding appropriate level of exercise given his obesity and risk of heart disease.

Effects on Cardiac Rhythm—Internist/Cardiologist

Possible mechanisms of antipsychotic-induced QTc prolongation are discussed in the following two sections.

Calcium Channel-Blocking Properties of Antipsychotic Medications

The interaction of antipsychotic medications with calcium channels remains an important but understudied issue. Many if not all antipsychotic medications increase QTc interval, reflecting a reduction in cardiac depolarization, corrected for cardiac rate (Welch & Chue, 2000). This is an important medical issue as antipsychotic administration can lead to sufficient QTc prolongation to increase the risk of significant cardiac arrhythmias including potentially fatal episodes of torsades de pointes (Belardinelli, Antzelevitch, & Vos, 2003). Therefore, psychiatrists often evaluate patients' ECG prior to initiation or change of a patient's medication. Although the rate changes secondary to antipsychotic exposure are well understood, as discussed in the following paragraph, little is known about mechanisms of inhibition of ventricular repolarization. However, older literature and a handful of more recent reports suggest that many antipsychotic agents act as calcium channel blockers, which may account for the cardiac complications (Buckley & Sanders, 2000; Christ et al., 2005; Enyeart, Dirksen, Sharma, Williford, & Sheu, 1990; Hatip-Al-Khatib & Bolukbasi-Hatip, 2002; Hull & Lockwood, 1986; Ishida et al., 1999; Kim, Tam, Siems, & Kang, 2005; Park et al., 2005; Prokopjeva, Barannik, Roshepkin, & Larionov, 1984; Qar, Galizzi, Fosset, & Lazdunski, 1987; Quirion, Lafaille, & Nair, 1985; Rochette-Egly, Boschetti, Basset, & Egly, 1982; Rojratanakiat & Hansch, 1990; Schaffer, Burton, Jones, & Oei, 1983; Schatzman, Wise, & Kuo, 1981; Thompson, Chen, Sample, Semeyn, & Bennett, 1986). There is also evidence that some antipsychotic agents, such as pimozide, block the rapid component, or $I(Kr)$, of the delayed rectifier potassium current, yielding electrophysiological effects similar to those of class III antiarrhythmic drugs (Drolet et al., 2001). Thus, it is important for internists and cardiologists to incorporate antipsychotic exposure when evaluating disorders of cardiac contractility, rate, and rhythm as well as choice of treatment.

Muscarinic AChR Antagonism and Antipsychotic Effects on Cardiac Rate

Antipsychotics increase cardiac rate. The usual risks from tachycardia are exacerbated by the presence of QT prolongation discussed above. Specifically, the combination of delayed cardiac repolarization with reduced interval to the next depolarization leads to the potential for overlay of depolarization on an already depolarized ventricle, the so-called torsades de pointes arrhythmia. This rate acceptation is generally attributed to direct anticholinergic, antipsychotic properties (e.g., clozapine, olanzapine, chlorpromazine) or addition of anticholinergic agents (benztropine) as a countermeasure for motor side effects that result from potent D_2 antagonists (e.g., haloperidol, risperidone). Muscarinic antagonism is thought to exert this effect by inhibition of the vagal input to the sinoatrial (SA) node (Eschweiler et al., 2002; Michelsen & Meyer, 2007; Mueck-Weymann et al., 2002). As noted above regarding development of QT prolongation, the presence of antipsychotic-induced tachycardia must be considered when choosing medications to slow heart rate. For example, propranalol is commonly prescribed to counteract the effects of antipsychotic-induced tachycardia. In this case, the SA node becomes relatively disconnected from both sympathetic and parasympathetic regulation. Thus, the patient is less able than usual to regulate heart rate in response to physiological stressors and metabolic requirements. The following clinical anecdote illustrates the risks and benefits of balancing antipsychotic treatment with cardiac risk.

Clozaril-Induced Tachycardia—Clinical Vignette

A patient in his early thirties was successfully treated with clozapine, achieving a moderate level of function and symptom remission. He was observed to have tachycardia (resting HR of 105–110) by his primary care physician. The physician was aware that clozapine is a highly potent muscarinic acetylcholine antagonist and advised the patient to discontinue clozapine in favor of an agent with lower propensity to increase heart rate. Although the tachycardia subsequently remitted, the patient relapsed with a protracted period of psychosis, hospitalization, and loss of function. Over the next 10 years the patient remained highly impaired, having lost his social contact and integration into his community. Thus, the decision to treat tachycardia without the awareness that Clozaril displays unique efficacy, resulted in tremendous harm to the patient's life course. An alternative approach would be to add propranolol or other beta blocker to control heart rate while considering overall risks and possibility of small reductions in Clozaril dose over several months while closely monitoring symptoms and function. In this case, a lack of appreciation for the overriding psychiatric risk and need to work with the patient's psychiatrist resulted in a very poor outcome.

Cardiac Conditions and Schizophrenia

Schizophrenia with Dilated Cardiomyopathy—CASE STUDY 6.5

Source: Patient, mother, and medical records.

History of present illness: The patient is a 25-year-old male who describes a 9-year history of difficulties dating back to high school. He states that at that time he changed from an honors student to having difficulty with memory and was unable to complete high school. He adds that this was in the context of substantial drug use as well as some alcohol. He describes prior use of LSD, marijuana, cocaine, and cough syrup. He and his mother state that he has been clean of all substance use for 5 years. The patient was initially treated with Trilifon, in 1992, which was augmented with lithium in 1993. He states he was then switched to Depakote after approximately 6 months and remains on this presently with improvement in mood swings. Olanzapine was initiated in approximately 1997 with improvement in symptoms as well as weight gain. The patient and his mother state that olanzapine was switched to quetiapine secondary to concerns over weight gain given his cardiomyopathy. However, the patient deteriorated on Seroquel, prompting initiation of clozapine in October 2000. He remains on 600 mg/day of clozapine, although he and his mother state that they have not seen improvement on this agent. Additionally, he was previously treated with Risperdal, which his mother states was moderately effective. She states that she requested that Risperdal be changed after she read that it could be associated with flashbacks from LSD use. They state he recently received a trial of haloperidol, up to 5 mg bid. His mother adds that she requested that it be discontinued after a NAMI (National Association for the Mentally Ill) newsletter that discouraged its use.* Additionally, he has taken fluvoxamine (Luvox) in the past. Neither he nor his mother recalls why it was discontinued. Additional medications include oxybutynin (Ditropan) for urinary incontinence and quinapril (Accupril) for familial dilated cardiomyopathy.

The patient states that his primary difficulties are recurrent thoughts of racial slurs that he finds disturbing as well as thoughts that others can read his mind or are trying to harm him. His mother adds that he checks the stove to make sure it is off repetitively throughout the day. He adamantly denies hallucinations, although his mother adds that he often asks her about comments he heard her make, yet she did not say. He currently attends a partial treatment program but has had to cut back due to concern that the people there could read his thoughts. He also states that he feels like he will be attacked at times but does not act to defend himself. He denies any current mood problems, and is without episodes of poor sleep or dangerous behavior.

Medical history: Familial dilated cardiomyopathy.

Medications: Depakote 2000 mg/day divided 1000 bid; olanzapine 20 mg/day divided 10 bid; clozapine 600 hs; Ditropan 20 mg/day; Accupril 20 mg/day.

Social history: He lives at home with his mother and reports no drug or alcohol use for 5 years. He drinks only decaffeinated coffee and quit smoking 5 days ago. He is unemployed.

Family history: His father died of a cardiac condition 19 years ago at the age of 37. His brother has dilated cardiomyopathy. A maternal

---

* There was a large amount of information disseminated through patient advocacy groups during this era suggesting benefit to new drugs. This phenomenon was perhaps due to associations with academic physicians that receive large amounts of money from drug companies. This story is an excellent example of how patients and their families were misled by so-called "thought leaders." For example, haloperidol is a very effective medication with low cardiac risk. It should not have been discontinued under these circumstances.

grandfather drank alcohol excessively and was in a psychiatric nursing facility in his later years.

Mental status exam:

Appearance and behavior: Pleasant 25-year-old man appearing his stated age.

Speech: Mildly pressured with normal volume.

Mood: Good.

Affect: Congruent and appropriate.

Thought process: Linear and goal directed.

Thought content: Remarkable for ideas of references regarding other peoples' actions and speech, as well as those of people in the media.

Perception: He denies perceptual abnormalities, although there is some evidence for auditory hallucinations, which he interprets as originating from people around him.

Insight and judgment: Good.

Assessment: Although the patient's presentation and diagnosis at age 16 was complicated by drug use, his current diagnosis is consistent with schizophrenia with strong affective and obsessive features. Despite a previous moderate response to olanzapine, he is currently experiencing a disabling exacerbation of obsessive thoughts and referential thinking with a high likelihood of hallucinations.

Recommendation: Taper to discontinue clozapine. Given the lack of efficacy and the side effects including nocturnal urinary incontinence, this agent is not clearly justified. Additionally, strong anticholinergic effects lead to a universal incidence of tachycardia with this agent, complicating its use in patients with existing cardiac abnormalities. Consider continuation of olanzapine during the Clozaril taper. However, olanzapine also has strong anticholinergic effects, which could affect heart rate. Ditropan may be discontinued as Clozaril is tapered because it is likely needed to counteract Clozaril-induced urinary incontinence. Continue Depakote, as this is the one medication they state has made a clear and sustained improvement.

Consider addition and possible switch to risperidone or halo-peridol because these agents would be best choices for high effi-cacy with low cardiac rate acceleration. The potential benefit of high-potency agents outweigh his mother's erroneous concern regarding the propensity of risperidone to cause flashbacks related to prior LSD. Consider reintroduction of Luvox, and titrate to 200 mg po bid to target obsessive symptoms.

Effects on Motor Systems—Internist/Neurologist

As noted in Chapter 1, patients with schizophrenia often manifest a host of motor abnormalities. Some of these difficulties, such as stiff-ness and akathisia, constitute true motor side effects of antipsy-chotic medication. However, many of the coordination difficulties and the late-onset choreiform movement called tardive dyskinesia are in fact manifestations of the illness rather than medication effects. Unfortunately, even many movement disorder specialists are unfamiliar with the motor manifestations of the illness and mistak-enly ascribe the problems to medication. Seizures are another albeit rare neurological concern for people with schizophrenia. Although all antipsychotic medications lower seizure threshold, this potential side effect is only problematic in practice with clozapine. Because seizure emergence is generally limited to cases in which the Clozaril level exceeds 1000 ng/mL, it is helpful to monitor Clozaril levels biannually or following escalation in dose. Interestingly, smoking causes a reduction in clozapine level, likely through interactions with hepatic metabolism via P450 enzymes. Therefore, smoking ces-sation is another potential precipitant to increased clozapine levels and should be considered when monitoring for seizure risk.

Effects on GI Motility and Liver Function—Gastroenterologist

Changes in Liver Function

Almost all antipsychotic medications are extensively metabolized by hepatic cytochrome P450 enzymes. Therefore, mild elevation of all liver enzymes can be expected. A new medication called 9-hydroxy-risperidone addresses this concern since it is the active metabolite of risperidone and is therefore "premetabolized." Since 9-hydroxy-risperidone is not extensively metabolized in the liver, it may be a better choice for patients with existing liver disease or who are on a large number of other medications that rely on hepatic degradation.

Constipation and Urinary Retention from Anticholinergic Medications

Several antipsychotic medications, most notably chlorpromazine, clozapine, and olanzapine, have a high degree of anticholinergic activity. Thus, these agents cause a variety of anticholinergic effects, most notably constipation due to reduced GI motility and urinary retention. Similarly, coadministration of anticholinergic medications such as benztropine to counter motor side effects results in the same effect.

7 ■ Emerging Targets and Non-Pharmacological Therapeutics

There are several new molecular targets that are being actively pursued. These include, but are not limited to, agents that facilitate N-methyl-D-aspartate (NMDA) receptor-mediated glutamate neurotransmission. Additionally, several investigators and pharmaceutical companies are investigating a possible role for full or partial agonists at a variety of nicotinic acetylcholine receptors including the alpha-7 homomeric subtype and alpha-4 beta-2 heteromeric receptors. Additionally, data from preclinical studies suggest that there may be a role for either phosphodiesterase inhibitors or erbB antagonists in future treatment of schizophrenia.

NMDA Agonists

There have been a number of clinical trials to examine the role for agents that facilitate NMDA receptor-mediated glutamate transmission. These agents include the amino acids glycine, serine, and d-cycloserine (Javitt, 2006; Javitt, Zylberman, Zukin, Heresco-Levy, & Lindenmayer, 1994; Rosse et al., 1989; van Berckel et al., 1999; Zylberman, Javitt, & Zukin, 1995). These amino acids bind to the allosteric facilitator glycine binding site to increase efficiency at the NMDA receptor. Despite being among the first truly novel treatments to emerge in 50 years, some data thus far have been disappointing (Figure 7.1) (Goff et al., 2005; van Berckel et al., 1999).

Nicotinic Agents

A number of preclinical studies have suggested that people with schizophrenia may have deficits in nicotinic acetylcholine receptor function. Among these, the largest body of literature has examined a possible role for agonists at the alpha 7-type nicotinic receptor (Adler et al., 2005; Freedman et al., 2006; Freedman et al., 2003;

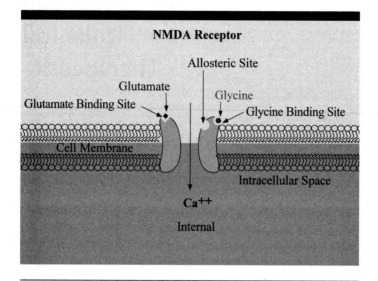

■ **Figure 7.1**   Stylized depiction of an activated NMDAR.

Stylized depiction of an activated NMDAR. Glutamate is in the glutamate binding site and glycine is in the glycine binding site. Allosteric sites that can modulate the receptor are shown in the unoccupied state. NMDA receptors require binding of two molecules of glutamate and two of glycine. For additional reading: Laube, B., Hirai H., Sturgess M., Betz H., & Kuhse J. (1997). Molecular determinants of agonist discrimination by NMDA receptor subunits: analysis of the glutamate binding site on the NR2B subunit. *Neuron, 18*(3), 493–503.

Simosky, Stevens, Kem, & Freedman, 2001). Future studies will examine whether or not these theoretical links, based largely on electrophysiological studies in animal models and patients, will translate to therapeutic benefit (Figure 7.2).

Phosphodiesterase Inhibitors

As noted above, there are convergent lines of evidence suggesting impairments in intracellular cAMP regulation in schizophrenia. The observation that all effective antipsychotic medications antagonize the dopamine D_2 G-protein-linked receptor, which itself inhibits cAMP formation, is among the most compelling of these arguments. Additionally, disruptions of cAMP formation in

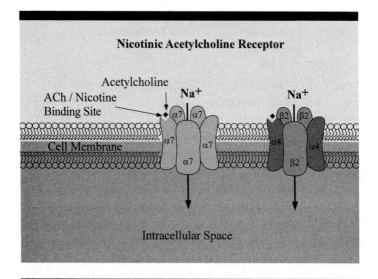

■ Figure 7.2   Stylized depiction of nicotinic acetylcholine receptor.

The nicotinic acetylcholine receptor is one of the main mediators of neurotransmission. This receptor is activated by the binding of acetylcholine, nicotine or agents that bind with relative selectivity to a subset of receptor subunits. As a ligand gated ion channel it permits the movement of positively charged ions from the synaptic cleft into the cytoplasm. Previous research suggested that agents binding homomeric alpha 7 (α7) receptors might provide cognitive benefits. However, recent preclinical and clinical data has not supported this idea. Alternatively, agents with selective affinity for alpha 4 beta 2 (α4β2) type receptors show greater promise as therapeutic agents for schizophrenia, cognition and smoking cessation.

animals recapitulates many phenotypic markers of schizophrenia including deficits in prepulse inhibition of startle, event-related potentials, as well as learning and memory (Gould et al., 2004; Kelly et al., 2007; Maxwell, Liang et al., 2006). However, recent studies have also begun to address alternative molecular targets to increase cAMP levels, including those responsible for cAMP degradation. For example, inhibitors of phosphodiesterases (PDE), which degrade cAMP, have been shown to meet several key criteria as antipsychotic agents in preclinical animal models (Kanes et al., 2007; Maxwell et al., 2004). Thus PDE inhibitors may present a new class of receptor-independent schizophrenia medications (Halene & Siegel, 2007) (see Figure 6.2 on page 142).

erbB Antagonists

Recent molecular genetic studies implicate an intracellular signaling protein called neuregulin 1 (NRG1) and its receptor, erbB, in the pathophysiology of schizophrenia (Stefansson et al., 2002; Stefansson, Steinthorsdottir, Thorgeirsson, Gulcher, & Stefansson, 2004). Among NRG1 receptors, erbB4 is of particular interest because of its crucial roles in neurodevelopment and in the modulation of N-methyl-D-aspartate (NMDA) receptor signaling. Furthermore, a recent study demonstrated alterations of NRG1-induced activation of erbB4 in the prefrontal cortex in schizophrenia using a postmortem tissue-stimulation approach (Hahn et al., 2006). This study found that NRG1 stimulation suppresses NMDA receptor activation in the human prefrontal cortex and that NRG1-induced suppression of NMDA receptor activation was more pronounced in schizophrenia subjects than in controls. These data suggest there may be enhanced NRG1-erbB4 signaling in schizophrenia and that enhanced NRG1 signaling may contribute to NMDA hypofunction in the disorder. This mechanistic linkage between NRG1-erbB signaling and NMDA receptor hypofunction further suggests that erbB antagonists may present a novel approach to alleviating symptoms or manifestations of schizophrenia that result from impaired NMDA receptor function (Figure 7.3).

mGluR2/3 Agonists

Recently, a family of compounds that stimulate metabotropic glutamate receptors type 2 and 3 (mGluR2/3) have shown efficacy for schizophrenia in small early-stage clinical trials (Patil et al., 2007) (Figure 7.4). At the time of publication of this book, it is not clear if this approach will ultimately prove effective. However, it constitutes the first new approach to schizophrenia in over 60 years, raising hope for iterative advances in treatment.

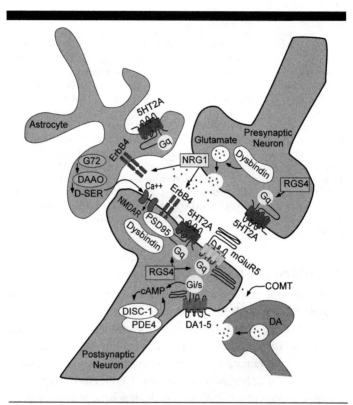

■ **Figure 7.3** Schematic representation of the inter-relationship among several of the proposed schizophrenia risk candidate genes.

Several of the relevant neurotransmitter systems (dopamine and glutamate) and signaling pathways (G-proteins, Neuregulin-ErbB4) are shown. Several of the recently proposed schizophrenia genes include COMT (catechol-O-methyltransferase), the enzyme that degrades dopamine at the synapse. Polymorphisms for COMT are linked to cognitive performance in schizophrenia and controls; DAAO (D-amino acid oxidase), is an endogenous co-agonist at the N-methyl-D-aspartate (NMDA) glutamate receptor; DISC-1 (disrupted in schizophrenia-1) is involved in axon growth and cortical development; dysbindin, (dystrobrevin-binding

(continues)

■ Figure 7.3 (continued)

---

protein 1), is localized to axon terminals and is associated with schizophrenia; NRG1 (neuregulin-1) is secreted by the presynaptic cell, binds the ErbB4 receptor on the postsynaptic cell and modulates activity of the NMDA receptor; G72 is a mitochondrial protein that has been linked to schizophrenia in some genetic association studies; PDE4 (phosphodiesterase 4) is the enzyme that degrades cAMP and acts in concert with dopamine receptor-linked G-Proteins to regulate intracellular cAMP levels; RGS4 (regulator of G protein signaling 4) has been linked to schizophrenia in some genetic association studies. Abbreviations: 5-HT^{2A} (serotonin receptor 2A), mGluR5 (metabotropic glutamate receptor 5), cAMP (cyclic adenosine monophosphate), DA (dopamine), DAR 1–5 (dopamine receptor types 1–5), D-ser (D-serine), ErbB4 (ErbB-type tyrosine kinase receptor B4), Glu (glutamate), Gq/Gi/Gs (Receptor-linked G proteins), NMDA (*N*-methyl-D-aspartate glutamate receptor), PSD95 (postsynaptic density protein 95). (Gray & Roth, 2007).

Nonadherence to Treatment

Medication nonadherence is the major risk factor for relapse and rehospitalization, with 55% of patients displaying significant difficulties adhering to treatment recommendations (Corriss et al., 1999). Nonadherent schizophrenia patients are twice as likely to undergo rehospitalization from relapse, resulting in a poor quality of life (Svarstad, Shireman, & Sweeney, 2001). For example, approximately 50% of schizophrenia patients relapse within 1 year of their latest episode, spending 15% to 20% of their time in psychiatric institutions (Ayuso-Gutierrez & del Rio Vega, 1997). Furthermore, the economic and social burden of healthcare costs for nonadherence in mental illnesses is estimated at $2.3 billion annually (Menzin, Boulanger, Friedman, Mackell, & Lloyd, 2003). Additional studies indicate that an actual medication adherence rate of 23% is in stark contrast to the patient-reported rate of 55%, while others find as few as 12% of patients achieve 1 year of uninterrupted antipsychotic medication (McCombs, Nichol, Stimmel, Shi, & Smith, 1999; Velligan, Lam, Ereshefsky, & Miller, 2003). Although many studies report medication adherence rates of 50%, it is increasingly thought that such data may be skewed, as many patients cease medication treatment once outside clinical trials

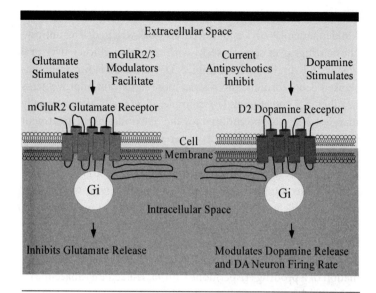

■ Figure 7.4 Metabotropic glutamate receptor type 2 (mGluR2) and dopamine D2 receptor (D2).

All current antipsychotic medications antagonize the dopamine D2 receptor, resulting in a reduction of the activity of an inhibitory G-Protein (Gi). This, intern causes disinhibition of Adneylyl Cyclase activity and an increase of intracellular cAMP. Changes in cAMP levels alter the activity of the enzyme PKA which alters a wealth of cellular functions including dopamine release and firing rate. A new class of medications in development, called mGluR2/3 positive allosteric modulators, binds to a modulatory site on mGluR2/3 autoreceptors of glutamatergic cells and facilitates the effects of glutamate. This enhances the activity of Gi, ultimately reducing release of glutamate. Clinical trials suggest these new agents may act as antipsychotic medications through a new mechanism.

(Seeman, 2001). This was recently demonstrated in the NIH-sponsored Clinical Antipsychotic Trials of Intervention Effectiveness (CATIE), where 74% of patients discontinued their medication despite being in a clinical trial (Keefe et al., 2005).

Use of Depot Preparations

Previous approaches to improve adherence through intramuscular administration were introduced in the mid-1960s and have proven effective (Blachly, 1965; Laffan, High, & Burke, 1965; McIlrath, 1967; Moldenhauer, 1966). Depot injections work well to deliver antipsychotic drugs over several weeks with enhanced efficacy over oral dosing (Adams, Fenton, Quraishi, & David, 2001). However, limitations of depot formulations restrict more significant improvements in adherence and efficacy. For example, adverse effects occasionally manifest and must be endured for the remainder of the treatment interval due to the inability to remove depot formulations. Prolonged pain often persists at repeated injection sites leading many patients to cease treatment (Bloch et al., 2001). Decanoate formulations are further limited by chemistry, with many compounds unable to form the ester linkage needed to make prodrug molecules. Recently, biodegradable microspheres made of polymers such as poly-lactide-co-glycolide (PLGA) have been used to administer a biweekly formulation of risperidone that does not require formation of a prodrug (risperidone Consta, Janssen Pharmaceutica). Although this approach shows promise in controlled studies, injections must be administered biweekly, requiring 24 annual treatment decisions (Harrison & Goa, 2004; Martin et al., 2003). Despite early promise, it is not yet clear what effect such a short delivery interval will have on practical application of this technology since adherence rates in the real world are estimated to be substantially lower than those in well-funded, labor-intensive clinical trials (Visco, Weidner, Cundiff, & Bump, 1999). Thus, depot medications may not provide adequate sustained care to many patients.

Indications to Develop Antipsychotic Implants

To address the need for more sustained treatment adherence, new methods of long-term medication delivery have been investigated using implantable systems for the treatment of schizophrenia (Hans, Dan, Winey, Lowman, & Siegel, 2004; Siegel, 2005; Siegel et al., 2002). Implantable systems have the capability to optimize a medication's therapeutic properties, rendering treatments that are more safe, efficacious, and reliable (Dash & Cudworth, 1998). Less medication is required and side effects can be minimized. Implantable systems can also be removed by a physician in case of adverse side effects, offering a degree of reversibility not available with depot injections. Additionally, mandatory removal at the end of the delivery interval is eliminated with biodegradable systems, cutting in half the inherent invasiveness to the patient (Fischel-Ghodsian & Newton, 1993). Recent studies by the authors of this book also indicate that more than 40% of patients and 75% of family members favor implants as a mechanism to maintain long-term medication adherence and health (Dankert et al., 2008; Irani et al., 2004). Thus, long-term delivery systems that guarantee adherence to medication could offer a solution to the most intractable, yet addressable cause of poor outcomes in schizophrenia.

Consequences of Nonadherence—CASE STUDY 7.1

Source: Patient and his sister.

History of present illness: The patient is a 54-year-old male who was first hospitalized at 21 years of age while in college. At that time he was drinking alcohol excessively and reports that he was diagnosed with anxiety and depression. However, he was discharged after 1 month on the antipsychotic medication Prolixin and Cogentin, suggesting a diagnosis or at least treatment for schizophrenia instead. He is described as reclusive at that time by his family. He was discharged to live with a family member, which his sister describes as both "to help the family member" and alternatively because "he was acting oddly." He worked for about 6 months, after which he has been supported by disability compensation. He was treated for many years with Prolixin, which was eventually given as a depot formulation.

Medical history: He has a history of renal failure and Goodpasture's disease leading to dialysis and treatment with prednisone. His condition has apparently resolved. He also has hypertension and hyperlipidemia.

Social history: The patient was married at 31 years of age and had a daughter while in that relationship. Both he and his wife carried diagnoses of schizophrenia. Their daughter is estranged from him as well as other relatives, and is described as having difficulties of an unclear nature. The patient lives in a retirement community.

Psychiatric history: The patient has been hospitalized approximately 10 times over the last 30 years, most recently discharged a few months prior to this evaluation. His hospitalizations are generally a product of stopping his medication, resulting in a progression to odd behavior, strange beliefs, and hallucinations over several weeks. Records indicate he was taking risperidone Consta (2-week depot formulation) in the past.

Medication:

Haloperidol 5 mg AM and 10 mg PM
Risperidone 4 mg PM
Metoprolol 25 mg 2×/day
Cogentin 1 mg 3×/day
Prednisone 5 mg/day
Os-Cal daily
Procrit 10,000 units sc monthly
Lipitor 40 mg daily
Enalapril 10 mg daily

Family history: Patient was seen with his sister present in the room. She is extremely supportive and remains involved in his life. She is 3 years older than him.

Mental status exam:

Appearance: Normal grooming and hygiene, in age-appropriate clothing.
Behavior: Pleasant and cooperative.
Speech: Normal volume with reduced amount.
Mood: Neither elated nor depressed presently.
Affect: Blunted.
Thought process: Logical.
Thought content: No current delusions elaborated.
Perception: Denied current hallucinations.

Insight: Good; recognizes and acknowledges his repetitive pattern of medication discontinuation leading to relapse.

Judgment: Good presently; however, his history indicates that he will have a lapse in judgment leading to relapse every 3 years.

Cognition: Formal testing not conducted; no difficulties noted on gross exam.

Assessment: The patient is a 54-year-old man with schizophrenia. He displays the classical pattern of recovery and a brief period of stability, followed by medication nonadherence due to a lapse in insight and judgment, inevitably leading to relapse. This pattern will persist as long as he has the ability to stop his medications. Of note, he is taking two medications that are identical for all intents and purposes, haloperidol and risperidone. Records indicate he "failed" risperidone Consta at 25 mg/2 weeks. However, he apparently did well for years on prolixin decanoate.

Recommendations: The patient will do better on depot medication than any other treatment. Since he is already on haloperidol and is doing well, it would make the most sense to switch him to haloperidol decanoate and discontinue the oral haloperidol and risperidone. His combined haloperidol plus risperidone dose is equivalent to approximately 20 mg of haloperidol per day. Therefore, he should receive 100 mg of haloperidol decanoate every month in place of his oral doses.

Upon the initial dose he should remain on his current regimen for 1 week then stop the risperidone for 1 week, then reduce haloperidol by 5 mg/week such that he will be off oral medication by the time he receives his second monthly injection.

Since he lives in a retirement home, it may be possible to have his shots administered on site. If not, however, his physician could administer them at monthly visits. The key will be to mobilize his family the moment he misses a shot.

▪ Poor Insight with Poor Outcome—CASE STUDY 7.2

Source: Patient seen in the presence of his parents.

History of recent illness: The patient is a 24-year-old male seen for a consultation and diagnostic impression. He was accompanied by his parents for the interview. The interview was performed under the condition that the patient was not identified as the proband. Rather, he was told by his family that he was there as part of family counseling for the discord over his circumstances. Thus, the interview was limited in scope in the service of establishing rapport. The interview lasted approximately 90 minutes. The patient appeared to be a reliable historian, as he was invested in telling his story.

The patient states that he was well until approximately 2 years ago, at which time he dropped out of college and began working at a local store. While there, he was using marijuana on occasion but came to believe that the owner of the establishment was selling drugs and was the target of an assassination attempt. He authored his first article at that time and later believed that the same group of people that targeted his boss was trying to kill him. Subsequently, he wrote a letter to a friend about "the truth." He believes that the government has been trying to kill him ever since that letter was sent and that his apartment is bugged, with someone watching his every movement. Thus, he spends a great deal of effort shielding himself from assassinations. He believes there is an elaborate system in place in which every person on the street is either after him, or part of a secret society of people that he has never met, that are there to protect him.

Over the past year he has been hospitalized for psychotic symptoms twice, once voluntarily for 7 days and later on an involuntary commitment for 20 days. In both cases he refused to take medication due to poor insight and certainty that all of his delusions are real.

The patient states that he lost contact with all friends and is unable to work due to the recent events (delusional content). He also indicates that his parents are withholding information from him and are now part of the worldwide conspiracy against him. He became very agitated during the interview when discussing his parents' role and whether or not he could trust them. He has been breaking phones and televisions to stop the monitoring by the government.

Medical and developmental history: No medical problems, parents describe him as a happy child with lots of friends. He was diagnosed with "learning difficulties" in school, which is of unclear meaning other than that he was in special reading classes. He had no behavioral problems and was well liked by teachers and peers.

Psychiatric and medical history: The patient had no previous history of psychiatric or medical illness. He is not taking any medication presently due to lack of insight.

Family history: There is no known history of psychiatric diagnosis. He has two siblings, neither of whom have psychiatric symptoms thus far.

Social history: He lives alone in an apartment. He does not work presently and spends a great deal of time on the Internet. His parents tried to restrict his Internet access after he sent a series of inappropriate messages.

Mental status exam:

Appearance: Well groomed and appropriate for his age.

Behavior: Calm and cooperative, becoming agitated toward the end when I suggested that medication might help him deal with his delusional content.

Speech: Normal rate prosody and amount.

Mood: Frightened, anxious, and depressed.

Affect: Congruent with mood.

Thought process: Linear.

Thought content: He demonstrates systematized paranoid delusions with total penetration of psychotic content into every sphere of life. He has no active suicidal or homicidal ideation. He is defensive but denies plan to attack his perceived pursuers.

Perception: He denies AH or other perceptual abnormalities.

Insight: Extremely poor; he has no sense that there are more realistic explanations for his decline in function and beliefs.

Judgment: Poor; his decisions regarding both life trajectory and medication now severely limit his ability to function, and may have long-term consequences due to the progression of un-checked psychosis.

Assessment: The patient is a 24-year-old male with significant psychotic content, leading to decline in function and isolation over a 2-year period. He meets criteria for schizophrenia. Although he had prominent mood symptoms at onset according to records, the mood component is now grossly overshadowed by frank psychosis. Given the diagnosis of schizophrenia, initiating treatment as soon as possible is of the utmost importance.

Recommendations: First and foremost the patient needs to take antipsychotic medication. However, his complete lack of insight makes that unrealistic presently. Therefore, I believe the best course of action is to engage in a therapeutic relationship that is directed at gaining trust. Unfortunately, it may require more drastic consequences and/or interventions before he agrees to treatment.

Treatment: If he agrees to oral medication treatment, several recent studies and meta-analyses suggest using olanzapine > risperidone = perphenazine = haloperidol = trifluoperazine > quetiapine = aripiprazole = ziprasidone. Use of less effective medications will likely reinforce that his delusions are real due to relatively poor therapeutic response in most patients. Of all antipsychotic medications, Clozaril will be the most effective, but it is unrealistic to expect him to comply with the complex and difficult treatment plan on Clozaril at the onset of treatment.

Alternatively, a depot preparation is likely to provide the most consistent and reliable treatment and therefore therapeutic effect. Haloperidol decanoate (1 mL via a small needle monthly) is much better than risperidone Consta (3 mL via large needle every 2 weeks). However, Consta is appropriate if the patient will not agree to haloperidol.

Addendum: The patient continued to decline treatment, becoming increasingly disenfranchised from his family. Under such circumstances, many municipalities will not engage patients in forced treatment unless they present a clear and present imminent danger to themselves or others. This unfortunately leads to the very common situation in which families are forced to wait for the affected individual to either hurt someone or be hurt before anyone intervenes.

Psychotherapy

Supportive

Supportive psychotherapy is a form of talking treatment that literally supports the patient's strengths and helps him or her cope with issues in his or her life in order to reduce or resolve the psychiatric symptoms. This approach is useful for disorders such as depression and anxiety, especially when a patient is not capable of accepting insight-oriented or cognitive therapies that require a more sophisticated interaction and patient effort. Among all forms of psychotherapy, supportive therapy has the most realistic role as an approach for schizophrenia since patients generally lack insight, and their hallucinations and delusions are not amenable to reasoning used in cognitive therapy (see below). Supportive therapy in schizophrenia is not effective for primary positive, negative, or cognitive symptoms. Rather, it is targeted at helping patients deal with their real-world problems of isolation and poor social and occupational function. Therapy in this context is similar to that in the treatment of cancer. That is, therapy can help the patients deal with their illness, but it is not the treatment for it.

Partial Hospital/Day Programs

Partial hospital programs, also called day treatment centers, are places where patients with severe psychiatric disorders can go for support, socialization, treatment, and literally, to have a place to go. The very existence of such centers illustrates the absolute severity of schizophrenia and the need for many patients to organize their entire existence around support services. By analogy, even severe medical disorders such as diabetes, coronary artery disease, and cancer do not require such a system to provide all-encompassing care.

Cognitive Behavioral Therapy

Cognitive behavioral therapy (CBT) is a form of psychotherapy that employs logical, evidence-based approaches to teach patients to evaluate their beliefs and resulting feelings. This technique is valuable in that it offers concrete goals and approaches to help patients address their problems. This approach was radical in its introduction in the early part of the last century because it offered a way for patients to progress rapidly toward resolution of an issue, rather than the pervading psychoanalytical approaches that required years of treatment without any specific goals or clear path. Recently, there have been some efforts to use CBT in schizophrenia. In the author's experience, this is unlikely to be a fruitful path. The nature of cognitive distortions in patients with schizophrenia is not amenable to logical analyses because they already accept ideas that defy all possible evidence. For example, a depressed patient may think that others do not like him or her. CBT allows the patient to evaluate the evidence in favor or refuting that supposition. For example, the patient may note the number of times a friend or family member has called him or her or sent a card as evidence that there are in fact people that like the patient. The resulting cognitive correction is then intended to alter the patient's self-image and mood. In schizophrenia, patients have beliefs that so far exceed reality that this approach is simply not effective. For example, a patient who believes that other people are putting thoughts into his or her head or that someone lives inside his or her head has already demonstrated that evidence and logic are not at play. In fact, one could say that "logic is not in the room" when discussing delusional content with schizophrenia patients. Furthermore, some patients will actually deteriorate if they are asked to recount and analyze their delusional content since this makes them focus on it, generally reinforcing their false beliefs.

Insight-Oriented Therapy

Most schizophrenia patients have a profound lack of insight into the reality of their situation. For example, a person who believes that there is a worldwide conspiracy against him or her has already forfeited any sense of introspection or ability to use evidence. As such, using insight-oriented approaches to help people with schizophrenia is similar to asking someone to cure a malignant tumor simply by understanding it.

Social Interventions

The most disabling aspect of schizophrenia results from the profound social isolation and societal disengagement that patients experience. Once an adult leaves the educational and vocational setting, there is little opportunity to meet other adults. The problem is further compounded by the fact that many patients suffer from poor motivation and a lack of social skills. Unfortunately, most programs that support social interactions for people with schizophrenia only provide contact with other psychiatric patients. This further reinforces the person's identity as a "psych patient." A number of programs, such as Compeer, do provide volunteer peers for people with major psychiatric illness. However well meaning, these programs still do not address patients' inability to meet other people on equal footing, the way they would in a professional or social situation.

Structured Environment

Patients with schizophrenia are often quite rigid and set in their ways. This mental inflexibility can be a weakness in situations that require adaptation such as a work environment that requires problem solving and finding solutions to new problems. However, people with schizophrenia will generally do better in environments that are constant and predictable. For example, tasks that do not vary day to day, or even hour to hour, will generally be more doable by people with schizophrenia than will jobs that constantly change. Similarly, a routine at home, with consistent meal times, medication regimens, and family schedules help people with schizophrenia manage a world that is always on the edge of being overwhelming.

Low Stress/Conflict

People with schizophrenia often react to stressful situations with psychotic exacerbations. This clinical observation is consistent with a variety of studies in animals showing that stress or stress hormones can recreate many of the biological abnormalities seen in schizophrenia patients. For example, there are characteristic EEG abnormalities in schizophrenia that can be recreated in mice that are treated with high-dose stress hormones. In patients this is manifested as psychotic exacerbations during times of change or high stress. For example, a patient may experience an increase in the amount and severity of hallucinations and delusions when family members are away, changing his or her routine and social support. Thus, it is critical to recognize that a stable, predictable, and low-stress environment will help people with schizophrenia remain at their best.

Electroconvulsive Therapy in the Context of Catatonia

Electroconvulsive therapy (ECT) is the most effective treatment to date for major depression. However, its role in schizophrenia is quite limited, if present at all. As noted in Chapter 1, a small percentage of schizophrenia patients experience catatonia, similar to that seen more typically in depression. For this population, and specific symptom, ECT may be indicated. However, ECT will only address the catatonia and is not an effective treatment for the more traditional symptom constellations of the disease. A few studies have started to examine the role of transcranial magnetic stimulation (TMS) for hallucinations. However, these investigations are in their infancy, and there is currently no evidence that anything but traditional dopamine antagonist antipsychotic medication can treat the positive symptoms of schizophrenia. Nothing to date treats the negative symptoms or cognitive deficits, and supportive therapy is likely to help patients navigate the real difficulties in their lives.

8 ■ Information for Specialties

Many people with schizophrenia have poor access to medical care, increasing the likelihood that they will present to nonpsychiatric practitioners with relatively late-stage or untreated illness. Additionally, there are aspects of schizophrenia that influence the etiology and/or treatment of nonpsychiatric diseases. Although the treating psychiatrist often functions as the primary care physician for this population, there are clearly instances in which an internist or specialist physician is required. This chapter describes how a diagnosis of schizophrenia is important to consider when treating nonpsychiatric conditions. For example, patients may ascribe early signs of illness to a psychotic explanation. Some patients may believe their pain emanates from someone putting items into their body or that the pain is being sent from another source. In such cases, a tumor or infection may go undiagnosed until it becomes sufficiently symptomatic that other people notice. Thus, physicians need to pay special attention with this population because the patients may either choose not to disclose or may not be capable of describing their symptoms. Other examples of how schizophrenia and its treatment are pertinent to various specialties are noted below. Clinical cases and vignettes are used to illustrate such instances.

Internist

In some instances, patients present to their primary care physicians with disorganization and odd behavior that threaten to complicate adherence to their medical treatment. Among these times, there are special circumstances in which it becomes critical to evaluate whether or not the psychotic component will have immediate adverse consequences for the patients and/or the people around them. For example, a person with tuberculosis must rigidly adhere to both medication and possibly isolation precautions during the infectious period. The following case report involves a woman that was seen for TB and immediately sent for a psychiatric evaluation to determine capacity to adhere to her medical regimen.

■ Patient Presenting with Tuberculosis—CASE STUDY 8.1

Source: Patient, her mother, and records from her internist.

History of present illness: Patient is a 48-year-old divorced black woman that was referred due to unusual behavior over the past 2 years. The patient was referred to her internist by the public health service after she was identified as having tuberculosis (TB). She is presently posttreatment for TB and continues in follow-up care with her internist. The patient presents today after seeing her internist earlier in the day. She was initially mute and appeared bewildered in the waiting room where she had been brought from her medical visit. The patient states she is here "to see if we need to get something together" and is unaware of what type of doctor I am or what type of problem is being evaluated. However, she readily agrees to evaluation after further discussion and explanation. Patient denies any problems. She states she is in the Navy and "between jobs," often referring to her platoon, driving planes, and her role in the government. She denies ever having actually piloted a plane and can offer no explanation for what she means by "enjoy driving planes." She is extremely vague and derailing with neologisms and with no apparent appreciation for the contradictory information she provides. She states she has seen a psychiatrist before, but cannot identify why, who, where, or when. Eventually she endorses that she may have been at another hospital 5 years ago, and has "heard of Risperdol," but not other psychotropic medications mentioned.

She describes herself as a loner throughout high school and states she was married for approximately 4 years at 21 years of age. She has had clerical jobs for "the government" as well as being a B5 in the Navy for the past 20 years, "on active duty" but not employed or doing anything for at least a year. She is unable to say how she passes her day other than "I like to be alone." She speaks with her family on a daily to weekly basis.

She endorses "interacting" with the TV and being able to read people's minds at times, and believes some people can read her mind. She denies perceptual abnormalities ever, and endorses "knowing" that she is under surveillance at times "in a car" or "on the street." She lived in a place with staff several years ago, but cannot explain where or why other than "for rest" and "they wanted me to." She refers to "them" and "they" often, but cannot elucidate who this refers to.

Her mother adds that the patient has been seen sitting and holding one-sided conversations, apparently responding to another participant. Also, her mother notes that the patient has never been in military. Rather, she last worked approximately 10 years ago and was well until her late 30s. Her mother also believes her husband was physically abusive, which she believes caused a traumatic miscarriage of the patient's only pregnancy. Her mother adds that the patient was admitted to a hospital 4 years ago and was discharged with a diagnosis of "depression or schizophrenia."

Past medical history: Tuberculosis, hypertension.

Medications: None.

Social history: Lives alone, unemployed on disability for TB, no drug or alcohol use, divorced 20 years prior, no children.

Family history: Both of her parents are alive. She has three sisters and four brothers with no known medical or psychiatric illnesses, according to the patient.

Mental status exam:

Appearance: Well groomed, well dressed.
Behavior: Pleasant and cooperative, no psychomotor agitation or retardation.
Speech: Low volume and reduced rate of speech.
Mood: "Good."
Affect: Appropriate but restricted.
Thought process: Derailing with neologisms; tangentiality and circumstanciality.

Thought content: Remarkable for beliefs of being under surveillance, "interacting with the TV and mind reading."

Perception: Denies perceptual abnormalities.

Insight: Very poor.

Judgment: Good; "I'll come see you and take medicine if you doctors think it will help me get back to school."

Assessment: Patient is a 48-year-old woman with signs of social and occupational decline with concurrent delusions and possibly hallucinations present since her mid 30s. Diagnosis consistent with schizophrenia—disorganized type. Tuberculosis does not contribute to her current mental status, as evidenced by symptoms 5 years earlier. It is important to consider her delusional content, which may affect her ability to conform to treatment guidelines for this highly infectious disease. Therefore, intervention with antipsychotic medication and increased social support and family vigilance are indicated.

Recommendation: Initiate trial of olanzapine for treatment of schizophrenia and tight monitoring for adherence to TB regimen by family members.

Dentist

Unfortunately, many patients with schizophrenia display very poor personal hygiene. This commonly manifests as resistance or simple negligence to attend to daily showers and oral care. The lasting consequences of the latter include a high proportion of schizophrenia patients having significant gum and tooth disease by middle age. Premature tooth loss and a high incidence of oral infections can ensue. Thus, special attention to oral care with annual visits to the dentist should be reinforced by family members.

Cardiologist

The unique issue faced in the schizophrenia population by cardiologists results from the cardiac side effects of antipsychotic medication. As noted earlier, virtually all antipsychotic medications cause QT prolongation (likely due to blockade of calcium channels) as well as rate acceleration. Together, these effects can cause QTc abnormalities, which can become dangerous when the absolute value for QTc exceeds 500 ms. As such, a person with schizophrenia that presents to a cardiologist with wide complex tachycardia may require a different treatment algorithm than a person with the same ECG pattern due to idiopathic causes.

Endocrinologist
Klinefelter's Syndrome

The following case presentation is relevant to the differential diagnosis between medical causes of psychosis and schizophrenia (Chapter 3). In such cases, it may be helpful to obtain a psychiatric consultation when first treating patients with cognitive, behavioral, or affective profiles that overlap with psychiatric conditions. However, the treating endocrinologist will be able to distinguish signs of schizophrenia from manifestations of the primary endocrinological disorder and treat all symptoms accordingly by adhering to the approach and criteria described below.

Klinefelter's Syndrome vs. Schizophrenia—CASE STUDY 8.2

Source: Patient with parents and records reviewed from his psychiatrist and prior neuropsychological testing.

History of present illness: Patient is a 40-year-old male who lives with his parents in a rural home. His parents have become increasingly frustrated with their son's behavior. Specifically, they report that he talks constantly in an uninterruptible fashion, becomes easily angered and upset, and is increasingly dependent upon them as well as isolated from his peers. He was adopted as an infant. He was told at a young age but did not accept this and became so upset that they "left it alone" at the advice of a treating psychiatrist. The patient was diagnosed with Klinefelter's syndrome at 16 years of age. He displayed delay in developmental milestones first noted at 4 months of age with motor difficulties and later by cognitive difficulties necessitating special education. He has never completed high school and currently functions at approximately a 4th-grade reading level according to records. Previous neuropsychological testing reveals a full IQ of 80 with a performance IQ of 88 and a verbal IQ of 74. The patient endorses that he has extreme difficulty with multiple tasks and is easily overwhelmed. He states that he does not take his antipsychotic medication (Loxitane) as it "sometimes makes my eyes go up and I could loose my hunting or driver's license." He expresses extreme frustration with his continued contact with the mental health system.

Past medical history: Klinefelter's syndrome.

Medications: Xanax 1 mg po qid prn, testosterone patch 5 mg/d, Loxitane—presently noncompliant.

Psychiatric history: Previously diagnosed with schizophrenia, depressive disorder, and dependent personality disorder. He has tried multiple antipsychotic as well as antidepressant medications including trifluoperazine, haloperidol, olanzapine, Loxitane, Luvox, Prozac, Klonopin, and Paxil by his report and records. His family states none have provided extended relief of symptoms.

Social history: Presently lives with parents, working at a nearby farm two afternoons per week. He is highly resistant to the idea of day treatment or independent/supported living outside the home. No history of drug use, remote social alcohol use, but no history of abuse. He has never been sexually active, has never had girlfriends or gone on dates.

Family history: Biological family unknown. His adopted brother died 7 years ago from HIV with a possible history of IV drug abuse. Both adoptive parents are seen by psychiatrists. His mother is treated with Paxil with good response and his father is treated with doxepin.

Mental status exam:

Appearance: Patient is a bearded 40-year-old male appearing his stated age with mild psychomotor agitation during interview.

Behavior: Without signs of behavioral control problems.

Speech: Rambling and increased amount but not pressured.

Mood: "Depressed."

Affect: Labile and tearful at appropriate times as well as irritable/angry when frustrated.

Thought process: Circumstantial.

Thought content: Lacks suicidal or homicidal ideation; no evidence of delusional content.

Perception: No abnormalities.

Insight: Limited regarding nature of difficulties; good regarding debilitating effects of Klinefelter's syndrome, "I have Klinefelter's. It's not good, but it's the way I was born, and it's the root of all of my problems."

Judgment: Fair.

Cognitively: Appears consistent with tested score of 80.

Assessment: 40-year-old male with Klinefelter's syndrome treated with testosterone, Xanax, and Loxitane. There is no evidence of comorbid schizophrenia. He also has extremely low frustration tolerance, with anxiety and depressive symptoms. His presentation is consistent with the psychiatric manifestations of his Klinefelter's syndrome with resultant cognitive limitations. As such, continued use of antipsychotic medication is not indicated.

Recommendations:

1. Supportive psychotherapy to target socialization and coping skills.
2. Day treatment or vocational rehabilitation program to help integrate him into a community. He is highly resistant to this idea.
3. Trial of an SSRI antidepressant targeting both anxiety and depressive symptoms. Specific recommendations include Zoloft 50 mg/day or Paxil working up to a dose of at least 40 mg/day.
4. Continue benzodiazepine with standing clonazepam to target resting anxiety rather than using intermittent Xanax.

Late-Onset Schizophrenia with Enlarged Thyroid—
CASE STUDY 8.3

Source: Patient, daughter, and records from the emergency room.

As noted previously, the coincident presentation of psychiatric and endocrinological symptoms raises the question as to whether or not a single etiology can account for all issues. The following case presentation describes an instance in which an enlarged thyroid and new-onset psychosis were detected at the same time in a middle-aged woman, raising the possibility that her primary endocrinological condition accounted for her psychotic symptoms.

Chief complaint: "Hearing voices for 1 year and concerned about people from the church around the corner trying to contact her through intercoms all over the city."

History of present illness: Patient is a 43-year-old female who describes 1 year of hearing voices that talk specifically to her over intercoms at work, in train stations, and throughout the city. She states that the voices began after she started working approximately 1 year ago. She had previously been a "welfare mom" raising four children, three sons of which (ages 14, 17, and 24) still live with her. She believes church members from a local church are angry at her because she "turned her life around" without them. She believes they are harassing her over intercoms. Her family has been aware of the voices over the past year. Both the patient and daughter say that the family originally thought, "It's no big deal, she's making it up or simply hallucinating." The patient's daughter now states she (the daughter) has come to realize that "The voices are real" and that the church people "really do" have an intercom system throughout the city to contact her mother. However, no one besides the patient has been able to hear the voices, despite the patient asking them to listen on multiple occasions. She presented to a local emergency department with a complaint of auditory hallucinations, at which time the ER physician noticed an enlarged thyroid. TFTs, Panel 7, CBC, and Utox were all normal at that time. Patient was transferred to a psychiatric emergency evaluation clinic, where the attending physician discharged her home with a script for Ativan 1 mg po qhs × 15 days for sleep. At her initial interview, the patient reported that voices went away while on Ativan and did not return since her visit to the ER. However, during a follow-up diagnostic interview a few days later, she disclosed that voices continued presently, and had not ever gone away. She also admitted that she told the psychiatrist that the voices were gone, and that she hadn't taken Ativan. She now believes people at church are coming up from a neighboring state, and that they will start harassing others once they're done with her.

Patient medical history: None, now with asymptomatic enlarged thyroid.

Psychiatric history: None.

Medication: None.

Family history: She denies any mental health issues in family with four children (oldest son with drug history and jail time; now clean for 3 years). She has 13 siblings. Of note, her family did not think hallucinating was problematic, and her daughter endorsed citywide conspiracy and intercom system. The patient is worried she's been having a "breakdown" since her father's death from cancer approximately 5 years ago.

Social history: On welfare until 1 year prior, when she began working in a cafeteria. Prior marijuana use (does not meet criteria for abuse)—no current use, "not in several years."

Data: Labs from prior ER visit without abnormalities. No record of brain imaging.

Mental status exam:

Behavior: Pleasant, cooperative.
Speech: Normal.
Behavior: No abnormalities.
Mood: Good.

Affect: Full and appropriate.

Thought process: Logical except in the sphere of delusions.

Thought content: Lacks suicidal or homicidal ideation; positive for marked delusions of conspiracy from church group.

Insight: Poor; "There is no way this could be my mind playing tricks on me. It's real."

Judgment: Fair, has not acted on delusions.

Assessment: Patient is a 43-year-old black woman with prominent auditory hallucinations and well-systematized delusion of church group trying to influence her via citywide intercom. Patient lacks any negative features of schizophreniform disorder—she is now at her highest level of occupational function ever achieved, and continues to care for three sons. No affective flattening or alogia; no mood component.

Plan: Initiate antipsychotic medication and refer to an endocrinologist for evaluation of enlarged thyroid.

Follow-up: The patient remained in psychiatric care with full resolution of psychiatric symptoms. Her enlarged thyroid was deemed noncontributory after full evaluation. As such, she received a diagnosis of schizophrenia and asymptomatic enlarged thyroid.

Urologist

Many psychiatric medications have anticholinergic effects. Some of these effects are peripheral to the intended action of the treatment (e.g., chlorpromazine, Clozaril, olanzapine), while others are used specifically as antidotes for motor side effects. In either case, urinary retention can be a disabling result, and patients often seek urological care. As such, it is imperative that simple steps, such as changing the psychiatric regimen, are considered prior to a urological workup or treatment. However, there are cases in which the psychiatric medication cannot be altered due to limited efficacy with other agents. This may well occur in a patient treated with olanzapine or Clozaril, the latter of which is arguably the best agent available. The following case illustrates how psychiatric treatment can result in urological consultation and intervention.

Urological Side Effects of Psychiatric Medications—
CASE STUDY 8.4

Source: Patient, husband, and son.

History of present illness: Patient was recently discharged from a local hospital after a 3-week inpatient admission for increasing persecutory ideation. The patient and family describe an abrupt onset of psychotic symptoms 14 years ago at age 40 during a family outing on a cruise. At that time the patient believed that another passenger was a detective who was trying to arrest her on drug charges. Additionally, she believed that waiters were trying to poison her and that the walls of her cabin disappear at night to allow people to poison her. She was committed for her first psychiatric hospitalization at that time and was treated with trifluoperazine for several years with good treatment response after which she stopped taking medications. Family states she continued without difficulties for a period of approximately 1 year until her second psychotic episode, at which time she believed she was accused of involvement in the murder of a local doctor she met one time. She was treated with haloperidol, initially by mouth, and later by depot due to poor compliance. Haloperidol depot provided her with significant symptom relief. The patient's husband states that as the years have passed, periods of remission become shorter and shorter until being interrupted by episodes of auditory hallucinations with persecutory ideation as stated above. Seven months ago the patient started olanzapine (10 mg hs), which was not helpful for 3 months. Quetiapine was added and titrated up to 400 mg daily for 2 months prior to her recent hospitalization. Haloperidol was added just prior to hospitalization. Additionally, she has been treated with Ativan, and valproic acid in the past. There is no history of suicidality.

During her most recent hospitalization, she was given Zoloft 50 mg qd for depressive symptoms, and Ativan was changed to clonazepam. She responded well to medications and left the hospital asymptotic on Benadryl, clonazepam 1 mg bid, Zoloft 50 mg qd, haloperidol depot 100 mg IM monthly, haloperidol 6 mg po bid, risperidone 4 mg po bid, Cogentin 1 mg po tid, and valproic acid 250 mg po bid.

Patient reports symptoms recurred approximately 1 week after haloperidol was decreased and eventually stopped, and valproate was decreased to 250 mg hs. After resumption of symptoms, haloperidol was reinitiated and titrated to 4 mg po tid. Patient developed severe tremor as well as urinary retention requiring initiation of Bethanocol from her urologist as well as Foley catheter placement.

Her symptoms now include persecutory ideation that people in her complex are detectives spying on her through electronic surveillance, that temporary tags on cars as well as "Christmas tree air fresheners" indicate the car of a detective. She experiences auditory hallucinations of detectives talking through the vents as well as the ceiling fan, to which she responds by yelling back at the fan. Additionally, she confronted a neighbor regarding the harassment and spying prior to hospitalization.

Medication:

Haloperidol depot 100 mg IM q month
Haloperidol 4 mg po tid
Cogentin 1 mg po tid
Depakote 250 mg po qhs
Risperidone 4 mg po bid
Zoloft 50 mg po qd
Bethanocol 10 mg po tid
Estradiol

Family history: Possible paternal aunt with mental illness, "reclusive and lived in institutions."

Social history: Lives with husband, no drug or alcohol use, formerly employed as a substitute teacher for approximately 3 years prior to onset of symptoms. After onset she stayed home and raised her children. She is a college graduate in 6 years over 4 universities, "I traveled around following my first husband, then got divorced and moved back home to attend college." She was remarried 1 year later at 21 years of age and had her first son at age 23. Her second son was born when she was 26 years old.

Developmental history: Patient indicates she "always had few good friends rather than many." She had normal performance throughout high school. In college she progressed from B's to A's and then C's for the last 2 years.

Past medical history: Hysterectomy.

Physical exam: Remarkable for severe bilateral tremor of the hands and legs with oral tremor of the lips and tongue.

Mental status exam:

Behavior: Patient is a pleasant cooperative female with normal speech.

Mood: "Good."

Affect: Flat (occasional smile).

Thought process: Logical.

Thought content: Positive for well systematized delusions of persecutory nature as previously stated. She presents with no suicidal or homicidal ideation.

Perception: Notable for auditory hallucination of voices emanating from fan and vents, as well as neighboring cars in traffic.

Insight: Limited: "It's real, not my brain playing tricks on me."

Judgment: Intact: "I would never harm anyone." Grossly without cognitive impairment, 30/30 on Mini Mental Status Exam.

Assessment: 54-year-old woman with psychosis marked by a 14-year history of recurring delusions of a persecutory nature, decline in social-occupational function, decreased interest in hobbies, intermittent auditory hallucinations, and ideas of reference. Her symptoms are consistent with the diagnosis of schizophrenia—paranoid type. Her age of onset is somewhat late but not exclusionary.

She is presently not responsive to polypharmacy with high-potency antipsychotics, and has marked extrapyramidal symptoms and urinary retention secondary to anticholinergic medication. She was previously nonresponsive to olanzapine and quetiapine.

Recommendation: Attempt to convert her current antipsychotic medications to Clozaril following an initial CBC with differential to screen for agranulocytosis. Long-term plan will be to slowly withdraw risperidone followed by oral haloperidol and eventually haloperidol depot. Immediate plan to discontinue Zoloft and valproate, as there is no clear indication for their continuation.

Immediate plan: Decrease risperidone to 2 mg po bid, and decrease Cogentin to 1 mg po bid. Anticipate that Bethanocol will be managed by urology with the expectation of discontinuation after Cogentin is tapered. Following CBC, initiate Clozaril at 25 mg po qhs with titration up by 50 mg per week to a goal of 200–400 mg po divided either qhs or bid (as tolerated) prior to discontinuation of haloperidol depot.

Gastroenterology (Gastroplasty)

Constipation due to anticholinergic properties is among the most common side effect of psychiatric medication. Usually, the effects are mild and can be managed with over-the-counter laxatives. Occasionally, however, it can become sufficiently problematic that patients need to change medications. The other complication involving the gastrointestinal system is weight gain secondary to increased appetite. Although this effect is mediated through changes in satiety centers in the CNS, it can become sufficiently severe that patients need to consider extreme measures such as gastroplasty. The following case illustrates one such example, in which the patient's poor impulse control, limited insight, and ambivalence (all symptoms of schizophrenia) affected his decisions regarding weight management and treatment.

Morbid Obesity Complicating Treatment of Schizophrenia—CASE STUDY 8.5

Source: Patient and family.

History of present illness: Patient is a 34-year-old male who presents without behavioral difficulties at this time. He is seeking recommendations for management of morbid obesity in context of schizophrenia. He and his family describe a 10-year history of intermittent medication noncompliance, each time resulting in deterioration leading to homelessness and self-neglect. However, during periods of compliance with medication, patient has generally done well, although not returning to previous level of function after each exacerbation. He had responded well to trifluoperazine for a period of several years, although over time he required change of medication. The patient lives in a residential care setting where he also receives psychiatric care from a nurse practitioner on a regular basis. He receives meals in the home as well.

Mental status exam:

Appearance: Pleasant, cooperative with exam.

Speech: Normal rate and tone.

Mood: Good.

Affect: Appropriate.

Thought process: Logical.

Perception: Denies hallucinations presently; however, does have them when noncompliant.

Thought content: No delusions at this time, but he admits to them during periods of noncompliance in the past. He denies any thoughts of either self-harm or harm to others.

Insight: Regarding psychiatric diagnosis, good.

Judgment: Good at this time.

There is no evidence of extrapyramidal side effects. Patient is morbidly obese and weighs 410 pounds at 5 feet, 8 inches, in height. His breathing is labored at rest although he is in no acute respiratory distress.

His mother states that he has consulted with nutritionists in the past, but has been unable to control his eating sufficiently to lose weight. He describes eating daily candy bars as a "snack" at his residence in addition to the meals served.

Medications:

Psychiatric medications being used are:

Risperdol 10 mg per day divided as 5 mg 2 × per day
Cogentin 1 mg 2 times per day
Quetiapine 150 mg before bed—recently added for irritability
Depakote 1000 mg 2 times per day—no history of seizures—added
    for behavioral control

Medical medications being used are:

Prevacid 30 mg per day
Furosemide 80 mg per day
Coreg 12.5 mg per day
Vasotec 10 mg per day
K-dur 80 mg per day

Assessment: 34-year-old male with clear history of schizophrenia and morbid obesity (over 400 pounds, 5′10″) that impairs his daily function. For example, he slipped and fell in a public restroom and was unable to lift himself off the floor. EMS was called; required four people to help him stand. Medications are likely to contribute to his weight gain, with Depakote as the most likely cause, and risperidone to a lesser extent. Additionally, the dose of risperidone he receives is sufficiently high to make it lose its so called "atypical" profile, leading to use of Cogentin as an adjunctive therapy for motor side effects. His additional medications are likely needed secondary to obesity.

Recommendations: Interventions for morbid obesity in the context of schizophrenia with extremely poor outcome including periods of aggression off medication are as follows:

1. Contact an eating disorders program with psychologists, psychiatrists, and other medical specialists that focus on a multidisciplinary approach to treat people with life-threatening obesity.

2. Depakote: Consider switching to Topamax for behavioral control, as this agent causes weight loss rather than weight gain. This change should occur under the supervision of a physician.

3. Risperidone: Consider switching to Moban, which is also thought to lack weight gain side effects. This too should be done under the care of a physician.

Follow-up: The patient transferred care to the evaluating psychiatrist. His medications were changed to trifluoperazine for control of psychosis and Topamax for behavioral control weight control. He remained without major psychotic exacerbations for the next 10 years, repeating the pattern of exacerbations only during limited periods of noncompliance. Despite changing to Topamax, he remained morbidly obese, leading to increasing cardiac, pulmonary, and endocrine problems including hypertension, sleep apnea, and insulin-dependent diabetes. He was referred for bariatric surgery, which he eventually declined. He was initially declined for the procedure secondary to concerns that he would be unable to comply with the postprocedure behavioral changes in eating pattern. Additionally, he was told that he was too obese for a reversible lap band procedure, which he favored over irreversible gastroplasty. Eventually, he was offered the procedure, but was cautioned that his medications would not fit into his reduced gastric capacity if taken on a twice-a-day schedule, necessitating him to take medications every 2 hours throughout the day to reduce the gastric burden. When given the opportunity to proceed with the procedure, the patient stated that he would lose the weight on his own without surgery, despite more than 15 years of clear failure to do so. Additionally, he was scared of surgery and declined to discuss it further when his family and physician noted that he was likely to suffer from increasingly serious medical morbidity due to his weight.

Surgery

The capacity to provide informed consent is among the most common issues related to schizophrenia that presents for surgeons. Although the vast majority of schizophrenia patients have capacity for such decisions, delusional content can sometimes intrude into this process. As in all medicine, this only becomes an issue when the patient's decision is at odds with his or her welfare. On such occasions, it can be helpful to engage a psychiatrist and family members to assess capacity and try to arrive at the appropriate balance of autonomy and benevolent intervention for the patient's health. Unfortunately, in many instances, the surgeon and related medical team cannot override the patient because the indicated procedure is not life-saving. The next clinical vignette illustrates how a patient's overarching delusions kept her from seeking indicated medical care despite her psychiatrist's strong urging to do so.

Refusal of Medical Care Secondary to Delusional Content— Clinical Vignette

The patient is a middle-aged, postmenopausal woman who believes that bugs live inside her and continually crawl out from her nose. She avoids contact with strangers and family alike so as to make sure she does not infect them with her bugs. Her delusional system has persisted throughout years of medication treatment. In addition to the loss of function and virtually total isolation that results from her, fear of infecting other people, she has persistently refused surgery to remove large fibroids that cause her pain and discomfort. She understands fully that she has fibroids, that they can be removed using laparoscopic procedures that will minimize risk to her, and that obtaining such a surgery would end her problem. However, she also believes firmly that she would infect the operating room once the incision was made, and the bugs would be able to escape freely. No degree of logic or treatment has swayed her. Since her fibroids are neither life-threatening nor urgent, there is no ability to override her decision even though it is completely baseless and rooted in psychotic content.

Gynecology

As noted above, psychotic content can intrude into important medical decisions such as surgical removal of large, painful fibroids. Additionally, psychosis can impede even routine gynecological care. For example, the following vignette illustrates how delusions can impede routine gynecological care.

Refusal of Treatment for a Urinary Tract Infection Due to Delusional Content—Clinical Vignette

The patient is a moderately obese 40-year-old woman who noted a foul-smelling odor emanating from her vagina. She added that the smell was accompanied by a bloody discharge. Her psychiatrist urged her to accept medication for a urinary tract infection or at least see her gynecologist for further evaluation. However, the patient was adamant that she did not have an infection, but rather that the imaginary woman that lives inside her and haunts her, was now causing the odor by putting things in her vagina. Again, in the absence of acute, emergent medical sequela, the psychiatrist is powerless to override her capacity and force treatment even though the decision is based purely on psychotic content. Similarly, she has refused to modify her diet or increase exercise because she believes it is the woman living inside her rather than adipose tissue that is causing her weight gain and increased girth. She will also not stop smoking since she believes it is the woman inside her rather than smoking that causes her to cough frequently.

9 ■ Family and Cultural Issues

Family Decision—What Does a Family Do When the Patient Will Not Accept Treatment?

What does a family do when the patient will not accept treatment or practice appropriate self-care? All too often, patients lack insight into their situation and refuse treatment as a result. In these tragic, albeit ubiquitous cases, families are forced to choose among bad and worse options. Many jurisdictions favor patient autonomy over health and safety. Thus, there is very little that can be done to force treatment on a sick individual, even when that sickness robs them of the basic comprehension of reality itself amid episodes of brain failure. This unjust, immoral, and inhumane situation likely stems from several factors. First, psychiatric illness was historically deemed a psychological condition, to be distinguished from "true" medical or neurological diseases. As such, the misunderstanding of the etiology of schizophrenia drove an approach in which the patient was seen as a product of poor parenting or practicing an alternative lifestyle. Despite overwhelming evidence that schizophrenia represents massive physiological, anatomical, and functional brain failure with virtually unparalleled morbidity across all of medicine, antiquated and misguided laws still retain the rights of psychotic individuals to throw away their lives based on hallucinations, delusions, and inability to comprehend the world around them. Because of these disgraceful laws, families must wait until patients actually harms themselves or someone else before the legal and medical systems can intervene and force hospitalization. Even in cases where the psychotic process results in harm, treatment is generally limited to a brief inpatient stay and may lack the authority to force pharmacological treatment.

In this context, many families are forced to embellish events leading up to a forced hospitalization in the service of obtaining humane psychiatric intervention. Such actions can only be seen as a sane reaction to an insane system that sacrifices their family member's health, safety, and future in the service of outdated, inaccurate, and barbaric laws. Privacy laws within the medical field also conspire to alienate families by allowing psychotic patients to direct who can be contacted and the extent to which family members may be engaged. This places the physician in a very awkward position of having to choose between the legal action and the ethical action. Certainly no one can dictate that physicians break the law in the service of humane medical intervention. However, one must always strive to frame schizophrenia as an illness of the family, to be managed by group decisions that keep the patients in continuous care such that they are able to appropriately participate in decisions that dictate their life outcomes.

Family Decision—Conflicting Priorities: Independence vs. Safety Net

Usually, families understand all too well the needs of the affected individual with schizophrenia. However, situations also arise in which the family's best intentions can impede the progress and well-being of the patient. One such situation arises from the conflicting needs for patients to integrate into society and be independent versus their need to receive social services and engage a safety net of support. Specifically, many families counsel patients not to seek full-time employment, lest they loose social security disability coverage for medical care and income. There is certainly merit to this argument, especially given the propensity of most patients to cease medication, relapse, and lose their jobs with frightening regularity. Thus, the most likely outcome if patients do obtain a full-time job is that they will lose benefits only to reapply later when they are (again) disabled. However, there is also a devastating consequence of this conservative approach. Patients remain isolated and demoralized without a "real" job. There are few, if any, opportunities for adults to meet peers outside of the work setting. Thus, patients that remain dependent on disability forfeit the ability to socialize outside of the psychiatric community. Although they may have interactions at day programs and drop-in centers, these relationships continue to reinforce their identity as a psychiatric patient. Alternatively, a job allows them to meet people as peers and develop a sense of self-worth based on contributions to a community.

Family Resources
Visions for Tomorrow

Visions for Tomorrow* consists of a series of workshops for direct primary caregivers of children and adolescents with brain disorders. Teachers of the program are trained family members who have experienced firsthand the rewards and challenges of raising children with brain disorders. The course offers caregivers an opportunity to share mutual experiences and learn valuable lessons from one another. The program covers educational material and provides the basics for day-to-day caregiving skills. The program has been widely disseminated and used by many National Alliance of Mental Illness (NAMI) state and affiliate offices across the country. The Visions for Tomorrow program has been used in over 28 states and by many NAMI state and affiliate leaders. The program continues to grow as NAMI state and affiliate leaders use it as a tool to reach families with children with mental illnesses.

For more information on the program, please visit the NAMI Texas Web site at http://texas.nami.org/VFT.htm.

Family-to-Family Educational Course

The NAMI Pennsylvania Family-to-Family Education Course is a free 12-week course, one evening per week, for family caregivers of individuals with severe brain disorders (mental illnesses). All instruction and course materials are free for class participants. The family-to-family curriculum focuses on schizophrenia, bipolar disorder (manic depression), clinical depression, borderline personality disorder, panic disorder, obsessive-compulsive disorder (OCD), and the dual diagnosis of mental illness together with

---

* Visions for Tomorrow was developed with support of the National Alliance of Mental Illness (Texas).

substance abuse. The course discusses the clinical treatment of these illnesses and teaches the knowledge and skills that family members need to cope more effectively.

One in four families have a relative suffering (some quietly) from a mental illness. The day-to-day struggles can be overwhelming. For close relatives of those with bipolar disorder (manic depression), major depression, borderline personality disorder, schizophrenia and schizoaffective disorder, panic disorder, obsessive-compulsive disorder, co-occurring brain disorders, and addictive disorders, a series of 12 weekly classes, once per week, is available that is structured to help family members understand and support their ill relative while maintaining their own well-being. The course is taught by a team of trained volunteer family members who know what it is like to have a loved one with a serious mental illness. There is no cost to participate in the NAMI family-to-family education program. Over 50,000 family members in the United States and Canada have completed this course.

Cultural Influence on Treatment

Different cultures interpret and treat mental illness differently. In some economically impoverished countries, psychotic reactions with paranoid delusions and hallucinations may be attributed to sorcery or witchcraft (Jilek & Jilek-Aall, 1970). Such episodes are characterized by confusion, emotional behavior, and cognitive deficits. Hence, these episodes have all of the hallmarks of a first-break episode of schizophrenia or bipolar disorder. In other cultures, such psychotic episodes may be seen as signs of weakness, to be treated with religious, rather than medical, interventions. Such cases can be challenging for the patients and their family as they are forced to confront long-held beliefs in the face of severe psychiatric illness that does not respond to nonpharmacological interventions, no matter how hard anyone tries to fit them into a culturally acceptable interpretation.

Cultural Influence on Family Interactions—Case Study 9.1
Source: The patient is a 23-year-old female college student. She was born in Asia, moved to the United States at 3 years of age and

then returned briefly to her home country, returning to the United States at age 5. Although the primary language in her home is not English, she describes English as primary for her. She denies any premorbid medical illnesses or psychiatric problems.

History of Present Illness: The patient states that she was lonely and anxious about making friends when she arrived at college but was initially able to handle courses in engineering at a highly competitive academic program. However, she took a leave of absence during her junior year secondary to psychiatric problems that she describes as "We say it was depression. My father saw the movie *A Beautiful Mind* and wanted me to just stop hearing voices." She later returned to school and made up two classes as well as "downgrading" her major to applied science. She received a *D* in a science class and an *A−* in her native language last semester. She is currently taking two classes and plans to complete her BA this semester. Her mother lives with her in college housing, and has done so since her return.

Initial symptoms included visual hallucinations of "blank pages" in a book her sister was reading, unintelligible words in a book she was trying to read, and odd clothing, "I was wearing my father's pajamas on one side and my mother's on the other." She also has referential religious and sexual delusions that are intertwined, "I can't look at people because my pastor said I have lust for power. I know he was talking directly to me because I was controlling him with my sexuality." She has stopped medication at times under the advisement of the Christian fellowship at her college, where an older student told her to discontinue care at student health in favor of praying. However, when her symptoms got worse, she resumed Zyprexa and Prozac under the care of student health. She states the Zyprexa makes the visual hallucinations and disturbing thoughts go away, but does not think the Prozac does anything. She thinks her religious convictions are consistent with her parents'. She also states that she believed that she had to be punished or repent for sins as a teenager, referring to normal developmental sexual thoughts and feelings. She has no friends or romantic relationships. She does not use any illicit drugs. She states she enjoys playing piano adding that she has a keyboard in her room, enabling her to play at any time. However, she does not ever do so. She eats all meals with her mother and states her mother accompanied her everywhere when she initially moved back to school last semester.

Other delusions include thinking that her college professor was reading her mind and telling her thoughts to the class during lecture and that other students were conspiring to harm her based on a comment in lab about "two tubes," which she was sure referred to something they were going to do to her body. She states she was very frightened at the time.

Mental status exam:

Behavior: No eye contact.

Speech: Very low volume, limited in amount initially with very long latency of response.

Mood: "Not depressed, just empty."

Affect: Flat, although she was eventually able to smile appropriately following empathetic engagement (my suspicion is that she does not change her facial expression without a skilled effort to illicit expression).

Thought process: Logical.

Thought content: Without suicidal or homicidal ideation, or current/new delusions, but clearly describes previous ones.

Perception: No current abnormalities.

Insight and Judgment: Patient's insight is good, "We call it depression;" clearly distinguishing her parents' wishes from the reality of her situation.

Judgment: Good; "They told me to stop treatment and just pray, but things got worse so I went back."

Assessment: 23-year-old Asian woman with schizophrenia—undifferentiated type. Although she has insight into her diagnosis and need for care, she is surrounded by significant supports that lack understanding and or insight. Both her family and social network made active attempts to disrupt appropriate medical care, albeit with good intentions. Ultimately, her prognosis is dependent on her family support. Therefore, the challenge in situations such as this is to engage the family and help them understand the distinction between faith and illness, as well as the reality of her needs.

Recommendation: She requires antipsychotic medication for life. She may need to shield this from her family and friends until they can be educated and/or engaged in her care.

Cultural Identity and Interpretation of First Break

The following vignettes were provided by a young woman with bipolar disorder and her close friend to provide two perspectives on a first psychotic break. As noted in the stories, the patient's cultural background played a large role in dictating her initial course of illness and her decisions.

Patient Perspective

I have experienced three psychotic breaks in the last 7 years. At the age of 20, I was diagnosed with manic bipolar disorder.

I had my first break after returning from a weeklong spring break trip to Haiti. I volunteered as a translator for a Catholic service group at the university I was attending. My parents were both born in Port Au Prince, Haiti, and I was born in New York City. I had traveled to the third world prior to this trip. However, I had never visited my parents' country of origin.

I observed the dichotomy of poverty and community. My experiences there opened my eyes to the misery and strife that the people faced daily. However, I also observed unity in this small village. A woman who had one child would feed her neighbor's children, not knowing what she was going to eat the next day. The people had faith in one another. Young children could safely visit each other alone. I saw a little girl who was no more than 3 years old telling her mom "good bye;" she was off to her friend's house.

I felt extremely relaxed in the central plateau of Haiti. I ate three meals a day, went to bed around 9 PM, and awoke when the cocks crowed loud enough to get me up, which was usually when the sun came up. My body was very connected and tuned in to the land. The most exciting part of the entire trip was being able to effectively communicate with the people and also acting as a bridge between the university students and the Haitian people.

Upon my return to the states I grew very depressed. However, it is only in retrospect that I recognize my state as depressed. I did not want to take the bus home from campus even though my apartment was about a mile and a half away; I walked daily, did not feel hungry, and stopped eating for an entire week. I cut off my shoulder length hair in an attempt to humble myself. I grew more and more unbalanced as each day passed, and it was difficult for me to sleep. I had a plethora of delusional thoughts. I believed that I needed to suffer as Jesus did and that the aftermath of this suffering would be ascension.

My weeklong episode ended with an arrest. I was angry at the United States because of what the non-governmental organization employees in Haiti told me about US policies. I was aimlessly walking around near my apartment complex and saw an American flag attached to a mailbox. I removed the flag from the mailbox and began to walk away with it. It was my small way of retaliating. The police were called, and I was arrested. I spent one day in prison. It was extremely difficult to be in a state of mania behind bars. My roommates and one of my university professors came and picked me up from the prison. The night I got back from the prison I was extremely paranoid. This was after 6 days of not eating or sleeping very much. Any small hole on the walls of my bedroom was perceived as a tiny camera watching my every move.

My family arrived the following morning. My sister and my dad immediately started to cry because I was in an extreme state of paranoia, I was about 20 pounds thinner and had very little hair on my head. My mother was a source of strength for me. She looked me in the eye and told me that I was going to get better. I believed her and agreed to go to the hospital that morning, and I stayed for one week. I was drugged so heavily that I didn't remember my dad saying goodbye to me. I arrived at the hospital on a Sunday and didn't really know where I was until Wednesday. I do remember getting rushed into the emergency room and having people look me in the eye and tell me that I would be okay. From Sunday afternoon through Wednesday is a blur. I was so manic that the doctors felt that my body needed to rest. My family told me that I did not spend the entire time sleeping; I watched television, and I went and saw the therapist daily; however, I do not recall any of this.

Upon my departure, I was given a prescription for 500 mg of Depakote and 3 mg of Risperdal. I was barely able to turn a doorknob under these medications. I was constantly hungry and sleepy. I was studying literature, and it took me about an hour to focus and read one page. Subsequently, I had to withdraw from some of my classes because I was unable to keep up. I continued to take the medication for about a month and then slowly weaned myself off.

I spent the summer completing the course work that I was unable to complete in the spring. I also took two summer courses, saw an on-campus therapist regularly and remained healthy my entire senior year. I graduated and took a position as a special education teacher in a high needs school. Two years after my first episode, I had another break.

Friends' Perspective

After asking a handful of Claudia's closest friends how they would describe her, you get a description using words like *compassionate, independent, grounded, charismatic, vivacious, empathetic,* and *fantastic listener.* No one would guess her story. On the outside she comes across calm and soothing. No one can tell the anxieties that twist in her head. She keeps them tied down and under control. It is on a rare occasion when she does not have it all in check that she gets overwhelmed, starts forgetting to sleep, forgetting to eat, and soon, if there is no one there to recognize her getting off track and to reel her in, there is no going back. Before she knows it she is in a full "episode" requiring the people around her to pull her out.

Claudia is the youngest of three daughters to a well-educated, hard working, Haitian family. Her father put all the kids through an all-girls private school and college while driving a cab in New York City. Claudia went from one of the largest cities in the world to a very rural college in central Pennsylvania. It was a culture shock, but she adjusted well with a tight group of friends. She earned a high GPA while majoring in English with diverse extracurricular activities.

Claudia has always considered herself Haitian, not American. Her stories are Haitian. The foods she eats are Haitian. Her family made sure she knew the difference growing up and felt it was important for her to hold onto her roots. So when her friends got together to go to her "mother" country she was right on board. She fell in love with Haiti. She said that you could *feel* the country while sitting on a hill in Haiti—that the distractions of billboards and media aren't there to confuse and interrupt your thoughts. She felt at home. The initial shock to her system came when she realized in Haiti she was no longer Haitian—she was American. It felt like her identity was being stripped away. Americans were stuck on appearance and lost track of themselves in material objects.

No one noticed how much she delved into her internal world until she came home to rural Pennsylvania. When she got back to college she felt even more disconnected from herself. She cut off her neatly woven locks of hair because she felt it was a sign of vanity. She left her apartment one day and started following buses around thinking they had special signs meant only for her. For example the *N* bus was telling her not to take it (*N* for *No*) while the *U* bus meant it was for her. Before she knew it, she was naked running in the street with an American flag she found in a housing development. She was arrested. While inside the cell, she stuck her head in the toilet to cleanse her shaven head. She thought Bob Marley was outside rioting to have her released. When her family arrived they were disappointed; they thought she was on drugs.

She thought they were on fire and continued to pour water on them to put them out. She was hospitalized and told she had a "brief psychotic episode." Her medication made her incredibly drowsy, and so, shortly after leaving the hospital, she stopped taking it. I met her a few months later.

When she told me the story, I was still convinced the piece of gum she chewed departing Haiti was laced with some long-lasting hallucinogen. Claudia was the most "normal" person I knew; fit, healthy, maybe smoked some marijuana on occasion, had a couple beers on a weekend night, but nothing out of the ordinary. She was going to succeed.

Claudia graduated and went directly into a master's program while teaching full time in one of the toughest schools in Brooklyn. She had an unconventional way of teaching, realizing that most of her students wouldn't get through high school, let alone college; she felt it was important for them to gain an understanding for the world outside of Brooklyn, so she had them read books like "Bridge to Terebithia" and taught them morals and a code of ethics to live by. She brought them on field trips to museums and brought in art projects. Her students did well, but she thought the other teachers thought poorly of her and started to make it more difficult for her to come to work by making her feel uncomfortable. Before long she had another "break." This time she wasn't in the hospital as long. Inside, she describes it as coming on more like a panic attack. On the outside she looked flat and sounded monotone and distant. They diagnosed her bipolar I with psychotic features and gave her more medications that she, again, became noncompliant with. She started to notice how her "episodes" erupted. She noticed it had to do with the structure of her life and that when she became stressed she would forget to eat and sleep on regular schedules. It wasn't long before she got back to herself. She found a boyfriend who understood and knew how to help her maintain balance.

It has been 5 years since her last episode. She is a behavioral analyst and teaches autistic children life skills. She continues to decline regular medication but will take a sedative on occasion when she becomes overwhelmed. Last month Claudia went to Colombia on her own. On the 12th day of her trip I received a message saying, "I have to find some malaria pills, we're going into the jungle." Eight days later I received an e-mail with misspelled words. "I had an episode. I didn't bring any medicine. I may need your help. It's not as bad as the first.—I'll call you when I get to Bogota." I soon found out she had been hospitalized and that her boyfriend and her sister were on their way to get her. Drugs were found in her body that she can't explain. She wants to stay in Colombia and is disappointed that her family wants her to leave. Right now she's too disconnected to write her own story, so I'm providing my perspective.

10 ■ Summary

Schizophrenia is among the most severe, debilitating, and devastating illnesses across all fields of medicine. It takes hold of individuals during late adolescence or young adulthood and dominates the remainder of their life course. Additionally, schizophrenia affects the patient's entire family and social structure owing to the pervasive nature of the disability and alternating course of remissions and exacerbation. Both genetic and environmental factors contribute to the risk for schizophrenia, although neither specific genes nor behaviors can be definitively linked to disease expression. All current medications treat the positive symptom cluster, including hallucinations, delusions, and disorganization. Unfortunately, none treat the negative or cognitive symptoms. Despite concerted efforts over the last two decades to create improved medications, it is now clear that antipsychotic medications have not changed in basic mechanism, dopamine D_2 receptor antagonism, since the invention of chlorpromazine in 1952. Accordingly, the prognosis for schizophrenia remains poor, with the majority of patients unable to fully integrate into either their former social or occupational roles. The future of medication development for schizophrenia remains unclear due to a dearth of well-established, validated targets. However, some efforts are focused on functional NMDA receptor agonists, nicotine receptor agonists, and modulators of intracellular cAMP levels. Additionally, interventions that increase adherence to medication, such as long-term delivery systems, are likely to have the greatest potential impact on improved outcome in schizophrenia in the near future.

References

Adams, C. E., Fenton, M. K., Quraishi, S., & David, A. S. (2001). Systematic meta-review of depot antipsychotic drugs for people with schizophrenia. *British Journal of Psychiatry, 179*, 290–299.

Adams, S. G., Jr., & Howe, J. T. (1993). Predicting medication compliance in a psychotic population. *Journal of Nervous and Mental Disorders, 181*(9), 558–560.

Addington, J., McCleary, L., & Munroe-Blum, H. (1998). Relationship between cognitive and social dysfunction in schizophrenia. *Schizophrenia Research, 34*(1–2), 59–66.

Adler, L. E., Cawthra, E. M., Donovan, K. A., Harris, J. G., Nagamoto, H. T., Olincy, A., et al. (2005). Improved p50 auditory gating with ondansetron in medicated schizophrenia patients. *American Journal of Psychiatry, 162*(2), 386–388.

Adler, G., & Gattaz, W. F. (1993). Auditory evoked potentials in schizophrenic patients before and during neuroleptic treatment. Relationship to psychopathological state. *European Archives of Psychiatry and Clinical Neuroscience, 242*(6), 357–361.

Adler, L. E., Olincy, A., Waldo, M., Harris, J. G., Griffith, J., Stevens, K., et al. (1998). Schizophrenia, sensory gating, and nicotinic receptors. *Schizophrenia Bulletin, 24*(2), 189–202.

Adler, L. E., Pachtman, E., Franks, R. D., Pecevich, M., Waldo, M. C., & Freedman, R. (1982). Neurophysiological evidence for a defect in neuronal mechanisms involved in sensory gating in schizophrenia. *Biology and Psychiatry, 17*(6), 639–654.

American Psychological Association. (2000). *Diagnostic and statistical manual of mental disorders* (4th ed., text revision). Washington, DC: Author.

Arango, C., Buchanan, R. W., Kirkpatrick, B., & Carpenter, W. T. (2004). The deficit syndrome in schizophrenia: Implications for the treatment of negative symptoms. *European Psychiatry, 19*(1), 21–26.

Arias Horcajadas, F. (2007). [A review about cannabis use as risk factor of schizophrenia]. *Adicciones, 19*(2), 191–203.

Ayuso-Gutierrez, J. L., & del Rio Vega, J. M. (1997). Factors influencing relapse in the long-term course of schizophrenia. *Schizophrenia Research, 28*(2–3), 199–206.

Bangalore, S. S., Prasad, K. M., Montrose, D. M., Goradia, D. D., Diwadkar, V. A., & Keshavan, M. S. (2008). Cannabis use and brain structural alterations in first episode schizophrenia—a region of interest, Voxel-based morphometric study. *Schizophrenia Research, 99*(1–3), 1–6.

Battle, Y. L., Martin, B. C., Dorfman, J. H., & Miller, L. S. (1999). Seasonality and infectious disease in schizophrenia: The birth hypothesis revisited. *Journal of Psychiatric Research, 33*(6), 501–509.

Belardinelli, L., Antzelevitch, C., & Vos, M. A. (2003). Assessing predictors of drug-induced torsade de pointes. *Trends in Pharmacological Science, 24*(12), 619–625.

Bellak, L., Kay, S. R., & Opler, L. A. (1987). Attention deficit disorder psychosis as a diagnostic category. *Psychiatric Development, 5*(3), 239–263.

Blachly, P. H. (1965). Depot fluphenazine enanthate treatment of outpatient schizophrenics. *Journal of New Drugs, 64*, 114–116.

Bloch Y., Mendlovic S., Strupinsky S., Altshuler A., Fennig, S., Ratzoni, G., (2001). Injections of depot antipsychotic medications in patients suffering from schizophrenia: do they hurt? *Journal of Clinical Psychiatry*, (62), 855–859.

Bona, J. R., Fackler, S. M., Fendley, M. J., & Nemeroff, C. B. (1998). Neurosarcoidosis as a cause of refractory psychosis: A complicated case report. *American Journal of Psychiatry, 155*(8), 1106–1108.

Boog, G. (2004). Obstetrical complications and subsequent schizophrenia in adolescent and young adult offspring: Is there a relationship? *European Journal of Obstetrics, Gynecology, and Reproductive Biology, 114*(2), 130–136.

Boutros, N. N., Belger, A., Campbell, D., D'Souza, C., & Krystal, J. (1999). Comparison of four components of sensory gating in schizophrenia and normal subjects: A preliminary report. *Psychiatry Research, 88*(2), 119–130.

Boutros, N. N., Korzyukov, O., Jansen, B., Feingold, A., & Bell, M. (2004). Sensory gating deficits during the mid-latency phase of information processing in medicated schizophrenia patients. *Psychiatry Research, 126*(3), 203–215.

Boutros, N. N., Zouridakis, G., & Overall, J. (1991). Replication and extension of P50 findings in schizophrenia. *Clinical Electroencephalography, 22*(1), 40–45.

Braff, D. L., Geyer, M. A., Light, G. A., Sprock, J., Perry, W., Cadenhead, K. S., et al. (2001). Impact of prepulse characteristics on the detection of sensorimotor gating deficits in schizophrenia. *Schizophrenia Research, 49*(1–2), 171–178.

Braff, D. L., Grillon, C., & Geyer, M. A. (1992). Gating and habituation of the startle reflex in schizophrenic patients. *Archives of General Psychiatry, 49*(3), 206–215.

Brodkin, E. S. (2005). Quantitative trait locus analysis of aggressive behaviours in mice. *Novartis Foundation Symposium, 268*, 57–69; discussion 69–77, 96–59.

Brodkin, E. S., Hagemann, A., Nemetski, S. M., & Silver, L. M. (2004). Social approach-avoidance behavior of inbred mouse strains towards DBA/2 mice. *Brain Research, 1002*(1–2), 151–157.

Browne, S., Clarke, M., Gervin, M., Waddington, J. L., Larkin, C., & O'Callaghan, E. (2000). Determinants of quality of life at first presentation with schizophrenia. *British Journal of Psychiatry, 176*, 173–176.

Buckley, N. A., & Sanders, P. (2000). Cardiovascular adverse effects of antipsychotic drugs. *Drug Safety, 23*(3), 215–228.

Carlsson, A., & Lindqvist, M. (1963). Effect of chlorpromazine or haloperidol on formation of 3-methoxytyramine and nor-metanephrine in mouse brain. *Acta Pharmacologica et Toxicologica (Copenhagen), 20*, 140–144.

Carpenter, W. T., Jr. (1994). The deficit syndrome. *American Journal of Psychiatry, 151*(3), 327–329.

Carpenter, W. T., Jr., Heinrichs, D. W., & Wagman, A. M. (1988). Deficit and nondeficit forms of schizophrenia: The concept. *American Journal of Psychiatry, 145*(5), 578–583.

Cheer, S. M., & Wagstaff, A. J. (2004). Quetiapine. A review of its use in the management of schizophrenia. *CNS Drugs, 18*(3), 173–199.

Christ, T., Wettwer, E., & Ravens, U. (2005). Risperidone-induced action potential prolongation is attenuated by increased repolarization reserve due to concomitant block of I(Ca,L). *Naunyn Schmiedebergs Arch Pharmacol, 371*(5), 393–400.

Clementz, B. A., Geyer, M. A., & Braff, D. L. (1998). Multiple site evaluation of P50 suppression among schizophrenia and normal comparison subjects. *Schizophrenia Research, 30*(1), 71–80.

Clementz, B. A., Keil, A., & Kissler, J. (2004). Aberrant brain dynamics in schizophrenia: Delayed buildup and prolonged decay of the visual steady-state response. *Brain Research. Cognitive Brain Research, 18*(2), 121–129.

Cooper, S. J. (1992). Schizophrenia after prenatal exposure to 1957 A2 influenza epidemic. *British Journal of Psychiatry, 161*, 394–396.

Corbett, R., Hartman, H., Kerman, L. L., Woods, A. T., Strupczewski, J. T., Helsley, G. C., et al. (1993). Effects of atypical antipsychotic agents on social behavior in rodents. *Pharmacology, Biochemistry, and Behavior, 45*(1), 9–17.

Correa, B. B., Xavier, M., & Guimaraes, J. (2006). Association of Huntington's disease and schizophrenia-like psychosis in a Huntington's disease pedigree. *Clinical Practice and Epidemiology in Mental Health, 2*, 1.

Corriss, D. J., Smith, T. E., Hull, J. W., Lim, R. W., Pratt, S. I., & Romanelli, S. (1999). Interactive risk factors for treatment adherence in a chronic psychotic disorders population. *Psychiatry Research, 89*(3), 269–274.

Cramer, J. R. (1998). Compliance with medication regimens for mental and physical disorders. *Psychiatric Services, 49*(2), 196–201.

Crawford, H. J., McClain-Furmanski, D., Castagnoli, N., Jr., & Castagnoli, K. (2002). Enhancement of auditory sensory gating and stimulus-bound gamma band (40 Hz) oscillations in heavy tobacco smokers. *Neuroscience Letters, 317*(3), 151–155.

Crow, T. J., & Done, D. J. (1992). Prenatal exposure to influenza does not cause schizophrenia. *British Journal of Psychiatry, 161*, 390–393.

Dankert, M. E., Brensinger, C. M., Metzger, K. L., Li, C., Koleva, S. G., Mesen, A., et al. (2008). Attitudes of patients and family members towards implantable psychiatric medication. *Schizophrenia Research* 105:279–286.

Dash, A. K., & Cudworth, G. C., 2nd. (1998). Therapeutic applications of implantable drug delivery systems. *Journal of Pharmacological and Toxicological Methods, 40*(1), 1–12.

Davis, J. M., Chen, N., & Glick, I. D. (2003). A meta-analysis of the efficacy of second-generation antipsychotics. *Archives of General Psychiatry, 60*(6), 553–564.

Delay, J., Deniker, P., & Harl, J. M. (1952). Therapeutic use in psychiatry of phenothiazine of central elective action (4560 RP). *Annals of Medicine and Psychology (Paris), 110*(2:1), 112–117.

Delay, J., Deniker, P., Harl, J. M., & Grasset, A. (1952). N-dimethylamino-prophylchlorophenothiazine (4560 RP) therapy of confusional states. *Annals of Medicine and Psychology (Paris), 110*(2–3), 398–403.

Dixon, L. B., Lehman, A. F., & Levine, J. (1995). Conventional antipsychotic medications for schizophrenia. *Schizophrenia Bulletin, 21*(4), 567–577.

Drolet, B., Rousseau, G., Daleau, P., Cardinal, R., Simard, C., & Turgeon, J. (2001). Pimozide (Orap) prolongs cardiac repolarization by blocking the rapid component of the delayed rectifier potassium current in native cardiac myocytes. *Journal of Cardiovascular Pharmacological Therapy, 6*(3), 255–260.

Eaton, W. W., Thara, R., Federman, E., & Tien, A. (1998). Remission and relapse in schizophrenia: The Madras Longitudinal Study. *Journal of Nervous and Mental Disorders, 186*(6), 357–363.

Enyeart, J. J., Dirksen, R. T., Sharma, V. K., Williford, D. J., & Sheu, S. S. (1990). Antipsychotic pimozide is a potent Ca2+ channel blocker in heart. *Molecular Pharmacology, 37*(5), 752–757.

Ereshefsky, L., Watanabe, M. D., & Tran-Johnson, T. K. (1989). Clozapine: An atypical antipsychotic agent. *Clinical Pharmacology, 8*(10), 691–709.

Erlenmeyer-Kimling, L., Rock, D., Roberts, S. A., Janal, M., Kestenbaum, C., Cornblatt, B., et al. (2000). Attention, memory, and motor skills as childhood predictors of schizophrenia-related psychoses: The New York High-Risk Project. *American Journal of Psychiatry, 157*(9), 1416–1422.

Erwin, R. J., Mawhinney-Hee, M., Gur, R. C., & Gur, R. E. (1991). Midlatency auditory evoked responses in schizophrenia. *Biology and Psychiatry, 30*(5), 430–442.

Erwin, R. J., Shtasel, D., & Gur, R. E. (1994). Effects of medication history on midlatency auditory evoked responses in schizophrenia. *Schizophrenia Research, 11*(3), 251–258.

Eschweiler, G. W., Bartels, M., Langle, G., Wild, B., Gaertner, I., & Nickola, M. (2002). Heart-rate variability (HRV) in the ECG trace of routine EEGs: Fast monitoring for the anticholinergic effects of clozapine and olanzapine? *Pharmacopsychiatry, 35*(3), 96–100.

Farde, L., Hall, H., Ehrin, E., & Sedvall, G. (1986). Quantitative analysis of D2 dopamine receptor binding in the living human brain by PET. *Science, 231*(4735), 258–261.

Farde, L., Wiesel, F. A., Jansson, P., Uppfeldt, G., Wahlen, A., & Sedvall, G. (1988). An open label trial of raclopride in acute schizophrenia. Confirmation of D2-dopamine receptor occupancy by PET. *Psychopharmacology (Berlin), 94*(1), 1–7.

Fenton, W. S. (2000). Prevalence of spontaneous dyskinesia in schizophrenia. *Journal of Clinical Psychiatry, 61*(Suppl 4), 10–14.

Fenton, W. S., Blyler, C. R., Wyatt, R. J., & McGlashan, T. H. (1997). Prevalence of spontaneous dyskinesia in schizophrenic and non-schizophrenic psychiatric patients. *British Journal of Psychiatry, 171*, 265–268.

Fenton, W. S., & McGlashan, T. H. (1994). Antecedents, symptom progression, and long-term outcome of the deficit syndrome in schizophrenia. *American Journal of Psychiatry, 151*(3), 351–356.

Fenton, W. S., Wyatt, R. J., & McGlashan, T. H. (1994). Risk factors for spontaneous dyskinesia in schizophrenia. *Archives of General Psychiatry, 51*(8), 643–650.

Firestone, P., & Peters, S. (1983). Minor physical anomalies and behavior in children: A review. *Journal of Autism and Developmental Disorders, 13*(4), 411–425.

Fischel-Ghodsian, F., & Newton, J. M. (1993). Analysis of drug release kinetics from degradable polymeric devices. *Journal of Drug Targeting, 1*(1), 51–57.

Freedman, R., Adler, L. E., Bickford, P., Byerley, W., Coon, H., Cullum, C. M., et al. (1994). Schizophrenia and nicotinic receptors. *Harvard Review of Psychiatry, 2*(4), 179–192.

Freedman, R., Adler, L. E., Waldo, M. C., Pachtman, E., & Franks, R. D. (1983). Neurophysiological evidence for a defect in inhibitory pathways in schizophrenia: Comparison of medicated and drug-free patients. *Biology and Psychiatry, 18*(5), 537–551.

Freedman, R., Leonard, S., Waldo, M., Gault, J., Olincy, A., & Adler, L. E. (2006). Characterization of allelic variants at chromosome 15q14 in schizophrenia. *Genes, the Brain, and Behavior, 5*(Suppl. 1), 14–22.

Freedman, R., Olincy, A., Ross, R. G., Waldo, M. C., Stevens, K. E., Adler, L. E., et al. (2003). The genetics of sensory gating deficits in schizophrenia. *Current Psychiatry Reports, 5*(2), 155–161.

Freeman, H. (1994). Schizophrenia and city residence. *British Journal of Psychiatry, Suppl*(23), 39–50.

Gallinat, J., Mulert, C., Bajbouj, M., Herrmann, W. M., Schunter, J., Senkowski, D., et al. (2002). Frontal and temporal dysfunction of auditory stimulus processing in schizophrenia. *Neuroimage, 17*(1), 110–127.

Geddes, J., Freemantle, N., Harrison, P., & Bebbington, P. (2000). Atypical antipsychotics in the treatment of schizophrenia: Systematic overview and meta-regression analysis. *BMJ, 321*(7273), 1371–1376.

Geyer, M. A., & Heinssen, R. (2005). New approaches to measurement and treatment research to improve cognition in schizophrenia. *Schizophrenia Bulletin, 31*(4), 806–809.

Geyer, M. A., Krebs-Thomson, K., Braff, D. L., & Swerdlow, N. R. (2001). Pharmacological studies of prepulse inhibition models of sensorimotor gating deficits in schizophrenia: A decade in review. *Psychopharmacology (Berlin), 156*(2–3), 117–154.

Goff, D. C., Herz, L., Posever, T., Shih, V., Tsai, G., Henderson, D. C., et al. (2005). A six-month, placebo-controlled trial of D-cycloserine co-administered with conventional antipsychotics in schizophrenia patients. *Psychopharmacology (Berlin), 179*(1), 144–150.

Gottesman, I. (1991). *Schizophrenia genesis: The origins of madness.* New York: Freeman.

Gould, T. J., Bizily, S. P., Tokarczyk, J., Kelly, M. P., Siegel, S. J., Kanes, S. J., et al. (2004). Sensorimotor gating deficits in transgenic mice expressing a constitutively active form of Gs alpha. *Neuropsychopharmacology, 29*(3), 494–501.

Gourion, D., Goldberger, C., Bourdel, M. C., Jean Bayle, F., Loo, H., & Krebs, M. O. (2004). Minor physical anomalies in patients with schizophrenia and their parents: Prevalence and pattern of craniofacial abnormalities. *Psychiatry Research, 125*(1), 21–28.

Gray, J. A., & Roth, B. L. (2007). The pipeline and future of drug development in schizophrenia. *Molecular Psychiatry, 12*(10), 904–922.

Green, M. F., Kern, R. S., & Heaton, R. K. (2004). Longitudinal studies of cognition and functional outcome in schizophrenia: Implications for MATRICS. *Schizophrenia Research, 72*(1), 41–51.

Green, M. F., & Nuechterlein, K. H. (2004). The MATRICS initiative: Developing a consensus cognitive battery for clinical trials. *Schizophr Research, 72*(1), 1–3.

Green, M. F., Satz, P., Gaier, D. J., Ganzell, S., & Kharabi, F. (1989). Minor physical anomalies in schizophrenia. *Schizophrenia Bulletin, 15*(1), 91–99.

Green, M. F., Satz, P., Soper, H. V., & Kharabi, F. (1987). Relationship between physical anomalies and age at onset of schizophrenia. *American Journal of Psychiatry, 144*(5), 666–667.

Gruen, P. H., Sachar, E. J., Langer, G., Altman, N., Leifer, M., Frantz, A., et al. (1978). Prolactin responses to neuroleptics in normal and schizophrenic subjects. *Archives of General Psychiatry, 35*(1), 108–116.

Gupta, S., Andreasen, N. C., Arndt, S., Flaum, M., Hubbard, W. C., & Ziebell, S. (1997). The Iowa Longitudinal Study of Recent Onset Psychosis: One-year follow-up of first episode patients. *Schizophrenia Research, 23*(1), 1–13.

Gur, R. C., Ragland, J. D., Moberg, P. J., Bilker, W. B., Kohler, C., Siegel, S. J., et al. (2001). Computerized neurocognitive scanning: II. The profile of schizophrenia. *Neuropsychopharmacology, 25*(5), 777–788.

Gur, R. C., Ragland, J. D., Moberg, P. J., Turner, T. H., Bilker, W. B., Kohler, C., et al. (2001). Computerized neurocognitive scanning: I. Methodology and validation in healthy people. *Neuropsychopharmacology, 25*(5), 766–776.

Guy, J. D., Majorski, L. V., Wallace, C. J., & Guy, M. P. (1983). The incidence of minor physical anomalies in adult male schizophrenics. *Schizophrenia Bulletin, 9*(4), 571–582.

Hahn, C. G., Wang, H. Y., Cho, D. S., Talbot, K., Gur, R. E., Berrettini, W. H., et al. (2006). Altered neuregulin 1-erbB4 signaling contributes to NMDA receptor hypofunction in schizophrenia. *Nature Medicine, 12*(7), 824–828.

Halene, T. B., & Siegel, S. J. (2007). PDE inhibitors in psychiatry-future options for dementia, depression and schizophrenia? *Drug Discovery Today, 12*(19–20), 870–878.

Hambrecht, M., Maurer, K., Hafner, H., & Sartorius, N. (1992). Transnational stability of gender differences in schizophrenia? An analysis based on the WHO study on determinants of outcome of severe mental disorders. *European Archives of Psychiatry and Clinical Neuroscience, 242*(1), 6–12.

Hans, M. L., Dan, L., Winey, K. I., Lowman, A. M., & Siegel, S. J. (2004). Daily to annual biodegradable drug delivery strategies for psychoactive compounds. In S. K. Mallapragada (Ed.), *Handbook of biodegradable polymeric materials & applications*. Stevenson Ranch, CA: American Scientific Publishers.

Harrison, P. J. (1999). The neuropathology of schizophrenia. A critical review of the data and their interpretation. *Brain, 122*(Pt 4), 593–624.

Harrison, T. S., & Goa, K. L. (2004). Long-acting risperidone: A review of its use in schizophrenia. *CNS Drugs, 18*(2), 113–132.

Hata, K., Iida, J., Iwasaka, H., Negoro, H. I., Ueda, F., & Kishimoto, T. (2003). Minor physical anomalies in childhood and adolescent onset schizophrenia. *Psychiatry and Clinical Neuroscience, 57*(1), 17–21.

Hatip-Al-Khatib, I., & Bolukbasi-Hatip, F. (2002). Modulation of the negative inotropic effect of haloperidol by drugs with positive inotropic effects in isolated rabbit heart. *Pharmacology, 66*(1), 19–25.

Ho, B. C., Andreasen, N. C., Flaum, M., Nopoulos, P., & Miller, D. (2000). Untreated initial psychosis: Its relation to quality of life and symptom remission in first-episode schizophrenia. *American Journal of Psychiatry, 157*(5), 808–815.

Hull, B. E., & Lockwood, T. D. (1986). Toxic cardiomyopathy: The effect of antipsychotic-antidepressant drugs and calcium on myocardial protein degradation and structural integrity. *Toxicology and Applied Pharmacology, 86*(2), 308–324.

Huntley, G. W., Vickers, J. C., & Morrison, J. H. (1997). Quantitative localization of NMDAR1 receptor subunit immunoreactivity in inferotemporal and prefrontal association cortices of monkey and human. *Brain Research, 749*(2), 245–262.

Huttunen, M. O., & Niskanen, P. (1978). Prenatal loss of father and psychiatric disorders. *Archives of General Psychiatry, 35*(4), 429–431.

Irani, F., Dankert, M., Brensinger, C., Bilker, W. B., Nair, S. R., Kohler, C. G., et al. (2004). Patient attitudes towards surgically implantable, long-term delivery of psychiatric medicine. *Neuropsychopharmacology, 29*(5), 960–968.

Ishida, H., Hoshiai, K., Hoshiai, M., Genka, C., Hirota, Y., & Nakazawa, H. (1999). Haloperidol prolongs diastolic phase of Ca(2+) transient in cardiac myocytes. *Japan Journal of Physiology, 49*(6), 479–484.

Ismail, B., Cantor-Graae, E., & McNeil, T. F. (1998). Minor physical anomalies in schizophrenic patients and their siblings. *American Journal of Psychiatry, 155*(12), 1695–1702.

Javitt, D. C. (2006). Is the glycine site half saturated or half unsaturated? Effects of glutamatergic drugs in schizophrenia patients. *Current Opinion in Psychiatry, 19*(2), 151–157.

Javitt, D. C., Zylberman, I., Zukin, S. R., Heresco-Levy, U., & Lindenmayer, J. P. (1994). Amelioration of negative symptoms in schizophrenia by glycine. *American Journal of Psychiatry, 151*(8), 1234–1236.

Jilek, W. G., & Jilek-Aall, L. (1970). Transient psychoses in Africans. *Psychiatric Clinics (Basel), 3*(6), 337–364.

Jin, Y., Potkin, S. G., Patterson, J. V., Sandman, C. A., Hetrick, W. P., & Bunney, W. E., Jr. (1997). Effects of P50 temporal variability on sensory gating in schizophrenia. *Psychiatry Research, 70*(2), 71–81.

Jonsson, H., & Nyman, A. K. (1984). Prediction of outcome in schizophrenia. *Acta Psychiatrica Scandinavia, 69*(4), 274–291.

Kane, J., Honigfeld, G., Singer, J., & Meltzer, H. (1988). Clozapine for the treatment-resistant schizophrenic. A double-blind comparison with chlorpromazine. *Archives in General Psychiatry, 45*(9), 789–796.

Kanes, S., Tokarczyk, J., Siegel, S., Bilker, W., Abel, T., & Kelly, M. (2007). Rolipram: A specific PDE4 inhibitor with potential antipsychotic activity. *Neuroscience 144*, 239–246.

Keefe, R. S. (2006). Neurocognitive effects of antipsychotic medications in patients with chronic schizophrenia in the CATIE trial. *Biology and Psychiatry, 59*(S), 965.

Keefe, R., Gu, H., Perkins, D., McEvoy, J., Hamer, R., & Lieberman, J. A. (2005). A comparison of the effects of olanzapine, quetiapine, and risperidone on neurocognitive function in first-episode psychosis. *ACNP Annual Meeting, 127*.

Kelly, M. P., Isiegas, C., Cheung, Y. F., Tokarczyk, J. A., Yang, X., Esposito, M. F., et al. (2007). Constitutive activation of $G_\alpha s$ causes deficits in sensorimotor gating due to PKA-dependent decreases in cAMP. *Neuropsychopharmacology 32*, 577–588.

Kendell, R. E., & Kemp, I. W. (1989). Maternal influenza in the etiology of schizophrenia. *Archives of General Psychiatry, 46*(10), 878–882.

Kendler, K. S., & Walsh, D. (1995). Gender and schizophrenia. Results of an epidemiologically-based family study. *British Journal of Psychiatry, 167*(2), 184–192.

Kim, E., Tam, M., Siems, W. F., & Kang, C. (2005). Effects of drugs with muscle-related side effects and affinity for calsequestrin on the calcium regulatory function of sarcoplasmic reticulum microsomes. *Molecular Pharmacology, 68*(6), 1708–1715.

Kinon, B. J., Stauffer, V. L., McGuire, H. C., Kaiser, C. J., Dickson, R. A., & Kennedy, J. S. (2003). The effects of antipsychotic drug treatment on prolactin concentrations in elderly patients. *Journal of the American Medical Directors Association, 4*(4), 189–194.

Kohler, C. G., & Martin, E. A. (2006). Emotional processing in schizophrenia. *Cognition and Neuropsychiatry, 11*(3), 250–271.

Kopala, L. C. (1996). Spontaneous and drug-induced movement disorders in schizophrenia. *Acta Psychiatrica Scandinavia Suppl, 389*, 12–17.

Koreen, A. R., Siris, S. G., Chakos, M., Alvir, J., Mayerhoff, D., & Lieberman, J. (1993). Depression in first-episode schizophrenia. *American Journal of Psychiatry, 150*(11), 1643–1648.

Lacro, J. P., Dunn, L. B., Dolder, C. R., Leckband, S. G., & Jeste, D. V. (2002). Prevalence of and risk factors for medication nonadherence in patients with schizophrenia: A comprehensive review of recent literature. *Journal of Clinical Psychiatry, 63*(10), 892–909.

Laffan, R. J., High, J. P., & Burke, J. C. (1965). The prolonged action of fluphenazine enanthate in oil after depot injection. *International Journal of Neuropsychiatry, 1*(4), 300–306.

Langer, G., Sachar, E. J., Gruen, P. H., & Halpern, F. S. (1977). Human prolactin responses to neuroleptic drugs correlate with antischizophrenic potency. *Nature, 266*(5603), 639–640.

Lastra, I., Vazquez-Barquero, J. L., Herrera Castanedo, S., Cuesta, M. J., Vazquez-Bourgon, M. E., & Dunn, G. (2000). The classification of first episode schizophrenia: A cluster-analytical approach. *Acta Psychiatrica Scandinavia, 102*(1), 26–31.

Lee, M. S., Kim, Y. K., Lee, S. K., & Suh, K. Y. (1998). A double-blind study of adjunctive sertraline in haloperidol-stabilized patients with chronic schizophrenia. *Journal of Clinical Psychopharmacology, 18*(5), 399–403.

Lewis, D. A., Hashimoto, T., & Volk, D. W. (2005). Cortical inhibitory neurons and schizophrenia. *Nature Reviews Neuroscience, 6*(4), 312–324.

Lewis, D. A., Volk, D. W., & Hashimoto, T. (2004). Selective alterations in prefrontal cortical GABA neurotransmission in schizophrenia: A novel target for the treatment of working memory dysfunction. *Psychopharmacology (Berlin), 174*(1), 143–150.

Lieberman, J. A., Alvir, J. M., Woerner, M., Degreef, G., Bilder, R. M., Ashtari, M., et al. (1992). Prospective study of psychobiology in first-episode schizophrenia at Hillside Hospital. *Schizophrenia Bulletin, 18*(3), 351–371.

Lieberman, J. A., Koreen, A. R., Chakos, M., Sheitman, B., Woerner, M., Alvir, J. M., et al. (1996). Factors influencing treatment response and outcome of first-episode schizophrenia: Implications for understanding the pathophysiology of schizophrenia. *Journal of Clinical Psychiatry, 57*(Suppl 9), 5–9.

Lieberman, J. A., Stroup, T. S., McEvoy, J. P., Swartz, M. S., Rosenheck, R. A., Perkins, D. O., et al. (2005). Effectiveness of antipsychotic drugs in patients with chronic schizophrenia. *New England Journal of Medicine, 353*(12), 1209–1223.

Loebel, A. D., Lieberman, J. A., Alvir, J. M., Mayerhoff, D. I., Geisler, S. H., & Szymanski, S. R. (1992). Duration of psychosis and outcome in first-episode schizophrenia. *American Journal of Psychiatry, 149*(9), 1183–1188.

Majewski-Tiedeken, C. R., Rabin, C. R., & Siegel, S. J. (2008). Ketamine exposure in adult mice leads to increased cell death in C3H, DBA2 and FVB inbred mouse strains. *Drug and Alcohol Dependence, 92*(1–3), 217–227.

Marder, S. R., Fenton, W., & Youens, K. (2004). Schizophrenia, IX: Cognition in schizophrenia-the MATRICS initiative. *American Journal of Psychiatry, 161*(1), 25.

Martin, S. D., Libretto, S. E., Pratt, D. J., Brewin, J. S., Huq, Z. U., & Saleh, B. T. (2003). Clinical experience with the long-acting injectable formulation of the atypical antipsychotic, risperidone. *Current Medical Research and Opinion, 19*(4), 298–305.

Maxwell, C. R., Ehrlichman, R. S., Liang, Y., Gettes, D. R., Evans, D. L., Kanes, S. J., et al. (2006). Corticosterone modulates auditory gating in mouse. *Neuropsychopharmacology 31*, 897–903.

Maxwell, C. R., Ehrlichman, R. S., Liang, Y., Trief, D., Kanes, S. J., Karp, J., et al. (2006). Ketamine produces lasting disruptions in encoding of sensory stimuli. *Journal of Pharmacology and Experimental Therapy, 316*(1), 315–324.

Maxwell, C. R., Kanes, S. J., Abel, T., & Siegel, S. J. (2004). Phosphodiesterase inhibitors: A novel mechanism for receptor-independent antipsychotic medications. *Neuroscience, 129*(1), 101–107.

Maxwell, C. R., Liang, Y., Kelly, M. P., Kanes, S. J., Abel, T., & Siegel, S. J. (2006). Mice expressing constitutively active G(s)alpha exhibit stimulus encoding deficits similar to those observed in schizophrenia patients. *Neuroscience 141*, 1257–1264.

Mayerhoff, D. I., Loebel, A. D., Alvir, J. M., Szymanski, S. R., Geisler, S. H., Borenstein, M., et al. (1994). The deficit state in first-episode schizophrenia. *American Journal of Psychiatry, 151*(10), 1417–1422.

McCombs, J. S., Nichol, M. B., Stimmel, G. L., Shi, J., & Smith, R. R. (1999). Use patterns for antipsychotic medications in Medicaid patients with schizophrenia. *Journal of Clinical Psychiatry, 60*(Suppl 19), 5–11; discussion 12–13.

McGlashan, T. H. (1999). Duration of untreated psychosis in first-episode schizophrenia: Marker or determinant of course? *Biology and Psychiatry, 46*(7), 899–907.

McIlrath, W. A. (1967). Experience with a depot phenothiazine in the treatment of schizophrenia. *Medical Journal of Austrailia, 1*(15), 760–762.

Megens, A. A., Niemegeers, C. J., & Awouters, F. H. (1992). Behavioral disinhibition and depression in amphetaminized rats: A comparison of risperidone, ocaperidone and haloperidol. *Journal of Pharmacology and Experimental Therapeutics, 260*(1), 160–167.

Meltzer, H. Y., & McGurk, S. R. (1999). The effects of clozapine, risperidone, and olanzapine on cognitive function in schizophrenia. *Schizophrenia Bulletin, 25*(2), 233–255.

Menzin, J., Boulanger, L., Friedman, M., Mackell, J., & Lloyd, J. R. (2003). Treatment adherence associated with conventional and atypical antipsychotics in a large state Medicaid program. *Psychiatric Services, 54*(5), 719–723.

Michelsen, J. W., & Meyer, J. M. (2007). Cardiovascular effects of antipsychotics. *Expert Review of Neurotherapeutics, 7*(7), 829–839.

Miller, A. L., Hall, C. S., Buchanan, R. W., Buckley, P. F., Chiles, J. A., Conley, R. R., et al. (2004). The Texas Medication Algorithm Project antipsychotic algorithm for schizophrenia: 2003 update. *Journal of Clinical Psychiatry, 65*(4), 500–508.

Moldenhauer, B. (1966). [Long-term therapy with depot-fluphenazine Dapotum in schizophrenia]. *Med Welt, 27,* 1477–1481.

Mueck-Weymann, M., Rechlin, T., Ehrengut, F., Rauh, R., Acker, J., Dittmann, R. W., et al. (2002). Effects of olanzapine and clozapine upon pulse rate variability. *Depression and Anxiety, 16*(3), 93–99.

Myhrman, A., Rantakallio, P., Isohanni, M., Jones, P., & Partanen, U. (1996). Unwantedness of a pregnancy and schizophrenia in the child. *British Journal of Psychiatry, 169*(5), 637–640.

Nordstrom, A. L., Farde, L., & Halldin, C. (1993). High 5-HT2 receptor occupancy in clozapine treated patients demonstrated by PET. *Psychopharmacology (Berlin), 110*(3), 365–367.

Nordstrom, A. L., Farde, L., Nyberg, S., Karlsson, P., Halldin, C., & Sedvall, G. (1995). D1, D2, and 5-HT2 receptor occupancy in relation to clozapine serum concentration: A PET study of schizophrenic patients. *American Journal of Psychiatry, 152*(10), 1444–1449.

O'Tuathaigh, C. M., Babovic, D., O'Meara, G., Clifford, J. J., Croke, D. T., & Waddington, J. L. (2006). Susceptibility genes for schizophrenia: Characterisation of mutant mouse models at the level of phenotypic behaviour. *Neuroscience and Biobehavior Review, 31*(1), 60–78.

Park, I. Y., Kim, E. J., Park, H., Fields, K., Dunker, A. K., & Kang, C. (2005). Interaction between cardiac calsequestrin and drugs with known cardiotoxicity. *Molecular Pharmacology, 67*(1), 97–104.

Patil, S. T., Zhang, L., Martenyi, F., Lowe, S. L., Jackson, K. A., Andreev, B. V., et al. (2007). Activation of mGlu2/3 receptors as a new approach to treat schizophrenia: A randomized phase 2 clinical trial. *Nature Medicine, 13*(9), 1102–1107.

Picton, T. W., & Hillyard, S. A. (1974). Human auditory evoked potentials. II. Effects of attention. *Electroencephalography and Clinical Neurophysiology, 36*(2), 191–199.

Picton, T. W., Hillyard, S. A., Krausz, H. I., & Galambos, R. (1974). Human auditory evoked potentials. I. Evaluation of components. *Electroencephalography and Clinical Neurophysiology, 36*(2), 179–190.

Plum, F. (1972). Prospects for research on schizophrenia. 3. Neurophysiology. Neuropathological findings. *Neuroscience Research Program Bulletin, 10*(4), 384–388.

Prathikanti, S., & Weinberger, D. R. (2005). Psychiatric genetics-the new era: Genetic research and some clinical implications. *British Medical Bulletin, 73–74*, 107–122.

Prokopjeva, V. D., Barannik, I. V., Roshepkin, V. Z., & Larionov, N. P. (1984). The influence of phenothiazines on the sarcoplasmic reticulum Ca-ATPase from skeletal and cardiac muscles. *Biochemistry International, 8*(6), 843–850.

Qar, J., Galizzi, J. P., Fosset, M., & Lazdunski, M. (1987). Receptors for diphenylbutylpiperidine neuroleptics in brain, cardiac, and smooth muscle membranes. Relationship with receptors for 1,4-dihydropyridines and phenylalkylamines and with Ca2+ channel blockade. *European Journal of Pharmacology, 141*(2), 261–268.

Quirion, R., Lafaille, F., & Nair, N. P. (1985). Comparative potencies of calcium channel antagonists and antischizophrenic drugs on central and peripheral calcium channel binding sites. *Journal of Pharmacy and Pharmacology, 37*(6), 437–440.

Rauser, L., Savage, J. E., Meltzer, H. Y., & Roth, B. L. (2001). Inverse agonist actions of typical and atypical antipsychotic drugs at the human 5-hydroxytryptamine(2C) receptor. *Journal of Pharmacology and Experimental Therapeutics, 299* (1), 83–89.

Remington, G. (2003). Understanding antipsychotic "atypicality": A clinical and pharmacological moving target. *Journal of Psychiatry and Neuroscience, 28*(4), 275–284.

Robinson, D., Woerner, M. G., Alvir, J. M., Bilder, R., Goldman, R., Geisler, S., et al. (1999). Predictors of relapse following response from a first episode of schizophrenia or schizoaffective disorder. *Archives of General Psychiatry, 56*(3), 241–247.

Rochette-Egly, C., Boschetti, E., Basset, P., & Egly, J. M. (1982). Interactions between calmodulin and immobilized phenothiazines. *Journal of Chromatography, 241*(2), 333–344.

Rojratanakiat, W., & Hansch, C. (1990). The relative dependence of calcium antagonists and neuroleptics binding to brain and heart receptors on drug lipophilicity. *Journal of Pharmacy and Pharmacology, 42*(8), 599–600.

Rosburg, T. (2004). Effects of tone repetition on auditory evoked neuromagnetic fields. *Clinical Neurophysiology, 115*(4), 898–905.

Rosenheck, R., Leslie, D., Keefe, R., McEvoy, J., Swartz, M., Perkins, D., et al. (2006). Barriers to employment for people with schizophrenia. *American Journal of Psychiatry, 163*(3), 411–417.

Rosse, R. B., Theut, S. K., Banay-Schwartz, M., Leighton, M., Scarcella, E., Cohen, C. G., et al. (1989). Glycine adjuvant therapy to conventional neuroleptic treatment in schizophrenia: An open-label, pilot study. *Clinical Neuropharmacology, 12*(5), 416–424.

Rummel, C., Kissling, W., & Leucht, S. (2006). Antidepressants for the negative symptoms of schizophrenia. *Cochrane Database Systematic Review, 3*, CD005581.

Schaffer, S. W., Burton, K. P., Jones, H. P., & Oei, H. H. (1983). Phenothiazine protection in calcium overload-induced heart failure: A possible role for calmodulin. *American Journal of Physiology, 244*(3), H328–334.

Schatzman, R. C., Wise, B. C., & Kuo, J. F. (1981). Phospholipid-sensitive calcium-dependent protein kinase: Inhibition by antipsychotic drugs. *Biochemical and Biophysical Research Communications, 98*(3), 669–676.

Schechter, M. D. (1980). Effect of neuroleptics and tricyclic antidepressants upon d-amphetamine discrimination. *Pharmacology and Biochemical Behavior, 12*(1), 1–5.

Sedvall, G. (1980). Relationships among biochemical, clinical, and pharmacokinetic variables in neuroleptic-treated schizophrenic patients. *Advances in Biochemistry and Psychopharmacology, 24*, 521–528.

Seeman, M. V. (2001). Clinical trials in psychiatry: Do results apply to practice? *Canadian Journal of Psychiatry, 46*(4), 352–355.

Seeman, P., Chau-Wong, M., Tedesco, J., & Wong, K. (1975). Brain receptors for antipsychotic drugs and dopamine: Direct binding assays. *Proceedings of the National Academy of Sciences, USA, 72*(11), 4376–4380.

Seeman, P., Corbett, R., & Van Tol, H. H. (1997). Atypical neuroleptics have low affinity for dopamine D2 receptors or are selective for D4 receptors. *Neuropsychopharmacology, 16*(2), 93–110; discussion 111–135.

Seeman, P., & Lee, T. (1975). Antipsychotic drugs: Direct correlation between clinical potency and presynaptic action on dopamine neurons. *Science, 188*(4194), 1217–1219.

Serper, M. R., Chou, J. C., Allen, M. H., Czobor, P., & Cancro, R. (1999). Symptomatic overlap of cocaine intoxication and acute schizophrenia at emergency presentation. *Schizophrenia Bulletin, 25*(2), 387–394.

Sham, P. C., O'Callaghan, E., Takei, N., Murray, G. K., Hare, E. H., & Murray, R. M. (1992). Schizophrenia following pre-natal exposure to influenza epidemics between 1939 and 1960. *British Journal of Psychiatry, 160,* 461–466.

Shen, W. W. (1999). A history of antipsychotic drug development. *Comprehensive Psychiatry, 40*(6), 407–414.

Siegel, S. J. (2005). Extended release drug delivery strategies in psychiatry: Theory to Practice. *Psychiatry 2005, 2*(6), 22–31.

Siegel, S. J., Irani, F., Brensinger, C. M., Kohler, C. G., Bilker, W. B., Ragland, J. D., et al. (2006). Prognostic variables at intake and long-term level of function in schizophrenia. *American Journal of Psychiatry, 163*(3), 433–441.

Siegel, S. J., Maxwell, C. R., Majumdar, S., Trief, D. F., Lerman, C., Gur, R. E., et al. (2005). Monoamine reuptake inhibition and nicotine receptor antagonism reduce amplitude and gating of auditory evoked potentials. *Neuroscience, 133*(3), 729–738.

Siegel, C., Waldo, M., Mizner, G., Adler, L. E., & Freedman, R. (1984). Deficits in sensory gating in schizophrenic patients and their relatives. Evidence obtained with auditory evoked responses. *Archives of General Psychiatry, 41*(6), 607–612.

Siegel, S. J., Winey, K. I., Gur, R. E., Lenox, R. H., Bilker, W. B., Ikeda, D., et al. (2002). Surgically implantable long-term antipsychotic delivery systems for the treatment of schizophrenia. *Neuropsychopharmacology, 26*(6), 817–823.

Simosky, J. K., Stevens, K. E., Kem, W. R., & Freedman, R. (2001). Intragastric DMXB-A, an alpha7 nicotinic agonist, improves deficient sensory inhibition in DBA/2 mice. *Biology and Psychiatry, 50*(7), 493–500.

Sivkov, S. T., & Akabaliev, V. H. (2003). Minor physical anomalies in schizophrenic patients and normal controls. *Psychiatry, 66*(3), 222–233.

Smits, L., Pedersen, C., Mortensen, P., & van Os, J. (2004). Association between short birth intervals and schizophrenia in the offspring. *Schizophrenia Research, 70*(1), 49–56.

Srisurapanont, M., Kittiratanapaiboon, P., & Jarusuraisin, N. (2001). Treatment for amphetamine psychosis. *Cochrane Database Systematic Review* (4), CD003026.

Stefansson, H., Sigurdsson, E., Steinthorsdottir, V., Bjornsdottir, S., Sigmundsson, T., Ghosh, S., et al. (2002). Neuregulin 1 and susceptibility to schizophrenia. *American Journal of Human Genetics, 71*(4), 877–892.

Stefansson, H., Steinthorsdottir, V., Thorgeirsson, T. E., Gulcher, J. R., & Stefansson, K. (2004). Neuregulin 1 and schizophrenia. *Annals of Medicine, 36*(1), 62–71.

Svarstad, B. L., Shireman, T. I., & Sweeney, J. K. (2001). Using drug claims data to assess the relationship of medication adherence with hospitalization and costs. *Psychiatric Services, 52*(6), 805–811.

Swerdlow, N. R., Braff, D. L., & Geyer, M. A. (2000). Animal models of deficient sensorimotor gating: What we know, what we think we know, and what we hope to know soon. *Behavioral Pharmacology, 11*(3–4), 185–204.

Swerdlow, N. R., Braff, D. L., Taaid, N., & Geyer, M. A. (1994). Assessing the validity of an animal model of deficient sensorimotor gating in schizophrenic patients. *Archives of General Psychiatry, 51*(2), 139–154.

Szymanski, S. R., Cannon, T. D., Gallacher, F., Erwin, R. J., & Gur, R. E. (1996). Course of treatment response in first-episode and chronic schizophrenia. *American Journal of Psychiatry, 153*(4), 519–525.

Szymanski, S., Lieberman, J. A., Alvir, J. M., Mayerhoff, D., Loebel, A., Geisler, S., et al. (1995). Gender differences in onset of illness, treatment response, course, and biologic indexes in first-episode schizophrenic patients. *American Journal of Psychiatry, 152*(5), 698–703.

Talbot, K., Eidem, W. L., Tinsley, C. L., Benson, M. A., Thompson, E. W., Smith, R. J., et al. (2004). Dysbindin-1 is reduced in intrinsic, glutamatergic terminals of the hippocampal formation in schizophrenia. *Journal of Clinical Investigation, 113*(9), 1353–1363.

Thakore, J. H. (2004). Metabolic disturbance in first-episode schizophrenia. *British Journal of Psychiatry, 47*(Suppl), S76–S79.

Thompson, D. P., Chen, G. Z., Sample, A. K., Semeyn, D. R., & Bennett, J. L. (1986). Calmodulin: Biochemical, physiological, and morphological effects on *Schistosoma mansoni. American Journal of Physiology, 251*(6 Pt 2), R1051–R1058.

Trichard, C., Paillere-Martinot, M. L., Attar-Levy, D., Recassens, C., Monnet, F., & Martinot, J. L. (1998). Binding of antipsychotic drugs to cortical 5-HT2A receptors: A PET study of chlorpromazine, clozapine, and amisulpride in schizophrenic patients. *American Journal of Psychiatry, 155*(4), 505–508.

Trixler, M., Tenyi, T., Csabi, G., & Szabo, R. (2001). Minor physical anomalies in schizophrenia and bipolar affective disorder. *Schizophrenia Research, 52*(3), 195–201.

Umbricht, D., Javitt, D., Novak, G., Bates, J., Pollack, S., Lieberman, J., et al. (1998). Effects of clozapine on auditory event-related potentials in schizophrenia. *Biology and Psychiatry, 44*(8), 716–725.

Valenstein, M., Copeland, L. A., Owen, R., Blow, F. C., & Visnic, S. (2001). Adherence assessments and the use of depot antipsychotics in patients with schizophrenia. *Journal of Clinical Psychiatry, 62*(7), 545–551.

van Berckel, B. N., Evenblij, C. N., van Loon, B. J., Maas, M. F., van der Geld, M. A., Wynne, H. J., et al. (1999). D-cycloserine increases positive symptoms in chronic schizophrenic patients when administered in addition to antipsychotics: A double-blind, parallel, placebo-controlled study. *Neuropsychopharmacology, 21*(2), 203–210.

van Os, J., & Selten, J. P. (1998). Prenatal exposure to maternal stress and subsequent schizophrenia. The May 1940 invasion of the Netherlands. *British Journal of Psychiatry, 172,* 324–326.

Velligan, D. I., Lam, F., Ereshefsky, L., & Miller, A. L. (2003). Psychopharmacology: Perspectives on medication adherence and atypical antipsychotic medications. *Psychiatric Services, 54*(5), 665–667.

Visco, A. G., Weidner, A. C., Cundiff, G. W., & Bump, R. C. (1999). Observed patient compliance with a structured outpatient bladder retraining program. *American Journal of Obstetrics and Gynecology, 181*(6), 1392–1394.

Wagman, A. M., Heinrichs, D. W., & Carpenter, W. T., Jr. (1987). Deficit and nondeficit forms of schizophrenia: Neuropsychological evaluation. *Psychiatry Research, 22*(4), 319–330.

Weiner, I. (2003). The "two-headed" latent inhibition model of schizophrenia: Modeling positive and negative symptoms and their treatment. *Psychopharmacology (Berlin), 169*(3–4), 257–297.

Welch, R., & Chue, P. (2000). Antipsychotic agents and QT changes. *Journal of Psychiatry and Neuroscience, 25*(2), 154–160.

Wyatt, R. J., Damiani, L. M., & Henter, I. D. (1998). First-episode schizophrenia. Early intervention and medication discontinuation in the context of course and treatment. *British Journal of Psychiatry, 172*(33), 77–83.

Yaktin, U. S., & Labban, S. (1992). Traumatic war. Stress and schizophrenia. *Journal of Psychosocial Nursing and Mental Health Services, 30*(6), 29–33.

Zylberman, I., Javitt, D. C., & Zukin, S. R. (1995). Pharmacological augmentation of NMDA receptor function for treatment of schizophrenia. *Annals of the New York Academy of Science, 757,* 487–491.

Key References

Diagnosis

American Psychiatric Association. (2000). *Diagnostic and statistical manual of mental disorders* (4th ed., text revision). Washington, DC: Author. This manual is the basis for diagnostic definitions and approaches used for psychiatric illnesses.

History of Antipsychotic Medication Discovery

Delay, J., Deniker, P., Harl, J. M., Grasset, A. (1952). N-dimethylamino-prophylchlorophenothiazine (4560 RP) therapy of confusional states. *Annals of Medicine and Psychology (Paris), 110*(2–3), 398–403. This is the first observation of successful pharmacotherapy of psychosis and provided the basis for all subsequent efforts to treat schizophrenia using a medical model.

Carlsson, A., & Lindqvist, M. (1963). Effect of chlorpromazine or haloperidol on formation of 3methoxytyramine and normetanephrine in mouse brain. *Acta Pharmacologica et Toxicologica (Copenhagen), 20*, 140–144. This study provided the earliest mechanistic understanding that all agents that effectively treat psychosis cause alterations in dopamine metabolism and turnover. As such, this finding allowed linkage to a particular neurotransmitter and eventually receptor systems that form the dopamine hypothesis of schizophrenia and psychosis.

Seeman, P., & Lee, T. (1975). Antipsychotic drugs: Direct correlation between clinical potency and presynaptic action on dopamine neurons. *Science, 188*(4194), 1217–1219. This study definitively establishes that all antipsychotic medications provide their effects via binding to the D_2 class of dopamine receptors, which remains true 30 years after its publication.

Medication Classification

Kane, J., Honigfeld, G., Singer, J., & Meltzer, H. (1988). Clozapine for the treatment-resistant schizophrenic. A double-blind comparison with chlorpromazine. *Archives of General Psychiatry*, 45(9):789–796. This paper demonstrated superiority of clozapine over other medications, allowing it to become the basis for a 25-year effort to replicate its superior efficacy and lack of motor side effects.

Geddes, J., Freemantle, N., Harrison, P., & Bebbington, P. (2000). Atypical antipsychotics in the treatment of schizophrenia: Systematic overview and meta-regression analysis. *BMJ*, 321(7273), 1371–1376. This is the first major publication to rigorously test widely held beliefs about the advantages of newer antipsychotic medications. This study showed that there are not significant advantages to newer agents, opening the door to subsequent studies corroborating this conclusion.

Remington, G. (2003). Understanding antipsychotic "atypicality": A clinical and pharmacological moving target. *Journal of Psychiatry and Neuroscience*, 28(4), 275–284. This article provides a systematic review of how the definition of *atypical antipsychotic* has changed over the past 15 years in recognition that previous definitions were not upheld.

Lieberman, J. A., Stroup, T. S., McEvoy, J. P., Swartz, M. S., Rosenheck, R. A., Perkins, D. O., et al. (2005). Effectiveness of antipsychotic drugs in patients with chronic schizophrenia. *New England Journal of Medicine*, 353(12):1209–1923. This landmark study provided a large multicenter, unbiased comparison of old and new medications and showed that newer agents do not demonstrate superiority to the older comparator medication.

Cognition in Schizophrenia

Gur, R. C., Ragland, J. D., Moberg, P. J., Bilker, W. B., Kohler, C., Siegel, S. J., et al. (2001). Computerized neurocognitive scanning: II. The profile of schizophrenia. *Neuropsychopharmacology*, 25(5),

777–788. This study describes qualitative and quantitative deficits across a broad range of cognitive domains in schizophrenia.

Motor Abnormalities in Schizophrenia

Fenton, W. S., Blyler, C. R., Wyatt, R. J., & McGlashan, T. H. (1997). Prevalence of spontaneous dyskinesia in schizophrenic and non-schizophrenic psychiatric patients. *British Journal of Psychiatry, 171*, 265–268. This publication is one of several by the lead author that dispel the widely held misconception that tardive dyskinesia (TD) is a medication-induced phenomenon. Rather, it clearly describes the evidence for motor abnormalities including TD as an integral part of schizophrenia.

Genetic Risk and Vulnerability Genes in Schizophrenia

Gottesman, I. (1991). *Schizophrenia genesis: The origins of madness.* New York: Freeman. This widely cited publication describes the genetic risk for relatives of individuals with schizophrenia. As such, it is one of the cornerstones for understanding the concept of genetic vulnerability in the illness.

Prathikanti, S., & Weinberger, D. R. Psychiatric genetics—the new era: Genetic research and some clinical implications. *British Medical Bulletin, 73–74*, 107–122. This article provides a snapshot of candidate genes for schizophrenia as well as an overview of how the field of psychiatric genetics has progressed over the last 5 years.

Neuroanatomical and Physiological Abnormalities in Schizophrenia

Lewis, D. A., Hashimoto, T., & Volk, D. W. (2005). Cortical inhibitory neurons and schizophrenia. *Nature Review of Neuroscience, 6*(4), 312–324. This review describes some of the most promising advances in neuroanatomical abnormalities in schizophrenia.

Freedman, R., Adler, L. E., Waldo, M. C., Pachtman, E., and Franks, R.D. (1983). Neurophysiological evidence for a defect in inhibitory pathways in schizophrenia: Comparison of medicated and drug-free patients. *Biology and Psychiatry, 18*(5), 537–551. This paper is among the initial descriptions of electrophysiological functional assays of neuronal abnormalities in schizophrenia.

Future Directions in Drug Discovery and Delivery

Siegel, S. J., Winey, K. I., Gur, R. E., Lenox, R. H., Bilker, W. B., Ikeda, D., et al. (2002). Surgically implantable long-term antipsychotic delivery systems for the treatment of schizophrenia. *Neuropsychopharmacology, 26*(6), 817–823. This paper introduces a novel approach to treating nonadherence to medication, which is the major determinant of outcome in schizophrenia.

Index

Italicized page locators indicate a figure; tables are noted with a *t*.